MW01145182

SWEET SUICIDE

SWEET SUICIDE

GENE WRIGHT

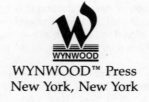

WYNWOOD™ Press
New York, New York

Library of Congress Cataloging-in-Publication Data

Wright, Gene, 1939–
   Sweet suicide.

   Includes bibliographical references (p.   )
   1. Sugar—Health aspects.   2. Nonnutritive sweeteners
—Health aspects.   I. Title.
QP702.S8W75   1989   613.2'8   89-24880
ISBN 0-922066-23-X

All rights reserved. No part of this publication may be reproduced, stored in a
retrieval system, or transmitted in any form or by any means—electronic,
mechanical, photocopy, recording, or any other—except for brief quotations in
printed reviews, without the prior permission of the publishers.

Copyright © by Gene Wright
Published by WYNWOOD™ Press
New York, New York
Printed in the United States of America

Contents

Foreword

THIS IS a book about sugar and sweeteners and their effects on the health of the mind and body.

It's no secret that within the last fifty years the consumption of sugar and other sweeteners in the United States has skyrocketed to astonishing levels. Since World War II these chemicals have been routinely added to an increasing number of foods and other products for reasons that have nothing to do with nutrition. Today, sugar and its sisters and substitutes are likely to be found in the majority of processed foods we eat, in the beverages we drink, and in the medicines we take.

Explaining why these substances are bad for you when taken in the massive amounts we consume them means also having to explain how and why we have come to develop such an insatiable sweet tooth. To unravel this complicated tale, I have taken a cross-cultural approach to the subject that cuts across the usual disciplines. Science in its narrowed vision of specialization generally fails to look at the larger picture or to place its investigations and conclusions in a societal context. Understanding the long-term effects on the human body of natural and artificial sweeteners requires a broader perspective than the one obtained by the usual scientific method of dissecting a problem into small, disparate elements.

At the basis of this study is a history of human nutrition and the inexorable invasion of sugar into the human diet. A knowledge of the past not only provides us with tools and warnings for the future;

it also serves as a point of entry into the investigation of sugar as a social and cultural phenomenon. Sugar is more than a product, it is a system. Through our repeated use, it has infiltrated our lives and developed its own protocols and usages, which are not confined to eating habits proper.

The central theme of this book is our failure to comprehend the untoward effects that have resulted from our ever-increasing reliance on fabricated, sweetened foods. The technology of food production and mass marketing and advertising techniques have subtly transformed our plentiful, nutritious foods into a sugar and chemical feast. The question of whether these new food technologies are clashing head first with human biology has largely been ignored by government agencies and major research groups. While the food industry pursues its own marketing interests, it blithely ignores the biological laws to which every living organism must adhere.

In explaining this phenomenon, I have drawn on the studies and conclusions of U.S. government agencies, consumer advocacy groups, and experts in the field of anthropology, sociology, medicine, psychology, and nutrition science. My intention is to provide the general reader who has an interest in good nutrition with information written in a nontechnical manner, and to provide the insights needed to avoid the pitfalls of a debased diet.

The human body is an amazingly resilient organism. Treated with respect and care, which means proper measures of food, relaxation, and work, it will serve you faithfully for years. But how healthy you will be—and how long you will live—depends largely on understanding what its requirements and limitations are. The cards may be stacked against you by our food manufacturers, but with the proper knowledge, and a little effort, you can free yourself from the eat sugar–want sugar syndrome that is at the heart of so many of the health problems of Americans today.

This book is dedicated to creating a healthier, more energetic, and more alert you.

G.W.
July 1989
New York City

SWEET
SUICIDE

1

Eat Now, Die Later

"Overeating destroys more than hunger."
—*Roman proverb*

TODAY, hunger and want are unknown to most of us who live in this generous, well-stocked larder called America. Scattered pockets of hunger persist among the homeless and chronically unemployed, but in general our high standard of living permits almost everyone to get an adequate and varied diet, whether at an expensive restaurant or a soup kitchen. For shoppers accustomed to the cornucopia of packaged goods available at supermarkets, it's impossible to imagine living as we did in the now-forgotten past, when our ancestors foraged and struggled daily tooth and nail in search of their next meager meal.

Yet, in achieving this welcome goal of boundless plenty, we have also managed to go nutritionally haywire. While our prehistoric ancestors had too little, today we have too much. That may be the most significant difference between us and them. They struggled to feed themselves; we struggle to resist the temptation of rich foods and excess calories. The sheer abundance of food in America has proved a mixed blessing that has left us in the paradoxical—and unprecedented—position of being both overfed and undernourished.

Although we've all been made aware of the link between nutrition and disease by health educators, the press, and government-sponsored advertising campaigns, too many of us still choose the wrong foods, and, to add injury to bodily insult, we consume more of these foods than our bodies can use or tolerate. We continue to ignore evidence that high blood pressure, heart disease, circulatory disease, kidney failure, cancer, and other ailments common to the Western World are related to what we eat and how much we eat. But one need only compare death rates compiled by the National Center for Health Statistics to food trends recorded by the U.S. Department of Agriculture to see that as our consumption of rich foods has soared during the last hundred years, so has the incidence of life-shortening diseases.

The chief players (and there are many minor ones) in our game of nutritional roulette are fats, salt, and sugars. None of these pose threats to health in themselves, and, except for artificial sweeteners, in balanced quantities they are essential to the proper functioning and repair of the body. Nutritional problems arise when we prefer them to the extent they displace foods we should be eating. That we have a taste for them is a fact not lost on the food industry, which does its best to see that we will continue to do so.

Fats: These give foods their flavor and impart the familiar satiated feeling we get after a heavy meal. As a result of public education on heart disease, many people have cut back on red meat, butter, and cheese (which contain saturated fats) in favor of fish, margarine, and imitation cheese made with vegetables oils (which are unsaturated). While there is evidence that unsaturated oils are better for you, the fact is that it doesn't matter what kind of fats you eat if you eat too much of them. Fats are fats and they all contribute to obesity and a host of other medical problems. The average American diet is still comprised of 37 percent to 50 percent fat,[1] or about twice the amount recommended by the Centers for Disease Control.

Salt: Sodium chloride enhances flavor and gives foods their "tang." Manufacturers use it as an inexpensive seasoning to "improve" the taste of inferior, overcooked, or overprocessed ingredients, ignoring the fact that salt can cause potassium imbalances and contribute to hypertension, at least in the amounts we ingest it. The National Academy of Sciences recommends from 1,100 milligrams to 3,000 milligrams of salt daily (about ½ to 1½ teaspoons), depending on how active we are, but most of us get a whopping 6,100 to 15,000 milligrams each day (about 3 to 5 teaspoons). Only a third of this amount is in the food itself; the remainder comes from processed and fast foods and by adding salt in cooking or at the table.

Sweeteners: Sugar in its many forms and low-calorie analogues imparts a sweet taste to foods that most people find desirable. The processed food industry finds them highly desirable too because they are an inexpensive means of getting consumers hooked on their products. While you are no doubt aware that soft drinks, candy, and many presweetened breakfast cereals are comprised primarily of sugar, you may be surprised to learn that sweeteners can be found in practically every manufactured product we put in our mouths. Sweeteners are in everything from frankfurters, bread, peanut butter, salad dressings, tomato sauces, horseradish, canned vegetables and soups, soy sauce, frozen TV dinners, wines, and liqueurs to vitamins, pain killers, antacids, mouthwashes, and toothpaste. For example, have you ever wondered why you prefer one brand of frozen vegetables over another? You may think that you buy the product simply because it tastes better, but a close inspection of the label will probably reveal that your preferred brand is the one with an added sweetener. Take a look around your kitchen and bathroom and check the labels. Sweeteners, you will find, are the food and drug industries' most common additives.

We Americans have been conditioned for decades to accept sugar and artificial sweeteners as a substitute for flavors that are routinely pulverized, pummeled, and percolated from our food supply. Through the manipulation of food technologists, our meals have been transformed into assembly-line products that, for all their convenience in preparation, would look, taste, and smell rather bland without the addition of colorings, sugar, salt, and other chemicals.

Food manufacturers know something most of us don't: that what we perceive as flavor has as much to do with our sense of smell as it does with our sense of taste. Although we have approximately 9,000 taste buds on our tongues (dogs have about 1,700; cats, 473), we taste only four basic food properties: sweet, salty, bitter, and sour or acid. Much more discriminating are our noses and their olfactory membranes, which can detect scents in dilutions as minute as one part in a billion. Flavor, then, is a complex perception involving not only taste but also the odor of food smelled through the nose and from inside the mouth as we eat; food seems tasteless when a head cold or inflamed sinuses impede these sensations.

Among the many ways manufacturers trick us into believing their products taste better than they do is the practice of "plating" instant coffee. Just before the jar is sealed on the assembly line, the coffee powder is sprayed with an aromatic coffee oil to give the illusion of fresh-brewed when the jar is opened. As anyone who has ever made a cup of instant coffee knows, the reconstituted coffee has little or no aroma. If you want flavor, you will have to add cream and sugar.

Putting the flavor back into factory-made food is the job of food chemists, who now know how to duplicate, or come close to, most natural flavors. A mixture of thirteen chemicals, for example, produces a reasonable facsimile of the flavor of cherries, thus allowing manufacturers to eliminate the real, and more expensive, fruit from its products. The synthetic flavoring is used primarily in soft drinks, most of which are nothing more than man-made chemicals in solution. In addition to the flavoring, a typical can of black cherry soda contains a coal tar dye, which imparts an unnatural, deep purple color, dispersants, acidulants, anti-foaming agents, preservatives, and, most of all, refined sugar and/or corn syrup or an artificial sweetener.

To "bring out" flavors— once an indication of wholesomeness—manufacturers use substances called flavor potentiators. How these work is not completely understood, but they seem to stimulate the flow of saliva which breaks down food and releases flavor. One of the most commonly used flavor potentiators is monosodium glutamate (MSG), an amino acid sprinkled into frozen dinners, canned soups, condiments, baked goods, and candy. Too much of this naturally occurring chemical can produce an allergic reaction, popularly known as the Chinese Food Syndrome for the reactions many experience after eating in Chinese restaurants that use MSG. Symptoms include excessive perspiration, flushing of the face, a feeling of numbness in the back of the neck and/or the arms, and general weakness. In 1969 the Food and Drug Administration (FDA) banned the use of MSG in baby foods (included to make the products taste better to mothers), after it was shown to cause brain damage in young laboratory animals.

The most popular flavor enhancers, however, are salt and sugar. Salt works best in warm, cooked products and snack foods, and has the added advantage, from the manufacturer's point of view, of creating a thirst for other products. Because a soft drink is cold and numbs the taste buds, more sugar is needed to intensify flavor and to produce the desired degree of sweetness. Sugar and salt, in fact, make up about 93 percent of the 150 pounds of food additives each of us eats every year.

Back in the 1970s, when the public first became aware of the dangers of sugar addiction, the Sugar Association mounted a massive advertising and public relations campaign to defend the food industry's common practice of adding sugar to products that don't need it. Sugar, affirmed an Association spokesperson in 1979, is "the catalyst that makes food eating pleasurable."[2] Barely seven years later, the Sugar Association cheered its acquittal by the Food and Drug Administration, which concluded, in a 229-page study of the health effects of sugar, that for people who consume a typical amount—equal to about 18 percent of daily calories—there "is no conclusive evidence that demonstrates a hazard."[3]

The FDA needn't have bothered, however, since in the interim the consumption of sugar had increased from 118 pounds annually per person in 1975 to more than 130 pounds today.[4] Some of us were obviously eating more than our allotted share, since the per capita consumption of sugar was presently 600 to 800 calories per day rather than the unrealistic 350 to 450 calories averaged by the FDA. One of the few important critics of the study was D. Mark Hegsted, former director of the Human Nutrition Center of the U.S. Department of Agriculture, who stated: "The report is accurate, but the conclusion is wrong. There is no advantage to high sugar consumption, nor is it likely that any will be found. As we encourage people to consume less fat, it would be a great mistake to replace those calories with sugar."[5]

While the FDA backtracked somewhat by characterizing its study as "an independent review, not an official document," the Sugar Association promptly ran full-page newspaper ads declaring, "Government Gives Sugar Clean Bill of Health." The effect of the highly publicized report was to assure the public it could now consume sugar at will. This perception was reinforced by the seeming indifference of the scientific establishment, the majority of whom had sanctified the correlation between dietary fat and heart disease while discounting evidence for the link between sucrose and coronary disease. Meanwhile, it was business as usual for the sugar industry, which was conjuring up ever new ways of putting sweeteners into our food supply.

Never mind that excessive consumption of sugar and sweeteners has been shown to contribute to hardening of the arteries, coronary thrombosis, cystic mastitis, yeast infections, irritable bowel syndrome, bladder and colon cancer, and a host of other diet-related ills. The medical establishment was on hand to rescue the unwary from the consequences of the food they eat. Our huge disease-treating apparatus—doctors, nurses, hospitals, miracle drugs, and intricate, life-sustaining machinery—will continue to offer the seriously ill a few extra weeks and months (although rarely years) of life. We look forward to new and better life-sustaining technologies to come, when in fact we have the means here and now to ward off many debilitating illnesses. The key, of course, is *prevention.* (The old saying, "An ounce of prevention is worth a pound of cure," has never sounded more compelling.) To stay healthy, we would be better off relearning lessons of the past than clinging to the promises of the medical future.

It wasn't until the fifth century B.C. that Hippocrates and other physicians came to the realization that food had something to do with good health. Medieval alchemists added to this kernel of nutritional knowledge by pointing out that some fruits and vegetables could also be used as medicines as well as poisons. Then, late in the eighteenth century, the French chemist Antoine-Laurent Lavoisier learned, while studying guinea pigs, that food is the body's fuel. All animals live by a kind of combustion process in which food is burned by oxygen, and carbon dioxide is given off according to amount of energy expended.

Lavoisier's pioneering work paved the way for later generations of researchers to identify the basic components of food: proteins, carbohydrates, and fats. By the 1920s, scientists had discovered that these basic foodstuffs contained other minute constituents essential to health: vitamins, minerals, amino acids, fats, and the like. While the body could make many of these nutrients from whatever food it was given, there remained more than forty others the body was unable to duplicate and which could be gotten only from food.

As a result, in 1941 the National Academy of Sciences began its campaign of Recommended Daily Allowances (RDAs) for the sixteen essential vitamins and minerals we should consume to stay in good health, to remain capable of reproduction, and to grow properly. These RDAs have since been adopted by many federal, state, and private nutritional programs. The brochures issued by these agencies usually feature attractive depictions of the foods we are supposed to consume daily, in their natural, unprocessed state: two servings of dairy products, four of cereal grains, four of fruits and vegetables, and two of meats and beans. The problem with this portrait is that it does not depict the foods we actually eat, nor does it depict these foods in the way they are often prepared. This classic approach to nutrition does not take into account all the substances that have been added to our food as it passes through the food manufacturers' assembly lines. Yet everything that goes into the body affects it in some way.

In a sense, we modern people are living in a biological time warp. Our Stone Age bodies must struggle daily with a twentieth-century diet to which they are poorly adapted. Although we owe our special place among all living things to our large brain and complex nervous system, we are physiologically not much different from the cavemen and cavewomen who preceded us. What has undergone a radical change is our environment and the foods we eat.[6] Within the 250 or so years since the Western World has undergone industrialization(a time span that is a drop in the evolutionary bucket), we have been eating more and more refined foods, and more and more substances have been added to our diets which are not found naturally on earth. These substances, like refined sugar, saccharin, aspartame, and hydrogenated fats, to name a few, are foreign to our systems.

Although our distant past is lost in the mists of history, we do know that our ancestors were omnivores who ranged woodland stretches and grasslands searching for whatever they could find or catch that was edible. These hunter-gatherers of the Paleolithic Age consumed a much greater variety of foodstuffs than we do today. Their cuisine consisted of ripe fruits, nuts, roots, grains, tender leaves and shoots, insects, lizards and frogs, and the occasional small mammal. Their menu might not be very tempting by contemporary standards, but it was rich in fiber, calcium, vitamin C, and other essential minerals and vitamins, and was low in saturated fats. Sugar came only as a complex carbohydrate contained in fruits and certain vegetables.[7] Honey was available as an occasional sweet, but gathering this precious liquid meant risking angry bee stings. In fact, the Stone Age diet closely follows the recommendations of today's nutritionists—and then some!

What our forebears ate is apparent from the structure of their— and our—teeth. We lacked the speed and strength of meat-eating predators and consequently never developed the large incisors that such animals as lions and tigers need to hold and kill their prey. To survive, we developed teeth that were more useful for chewing and grinding. Our facial structure has evolved into what it is today because our ancestors were primarily vegetarians who used their teeth to open shells, crack eggs, and break down the cellulose that most raw vegetation is comprised of. This primitive, relatively sugar-free diet accounts for the remarkable lack of tooth decay found in most fossils of the preindustrial past.

We can get a valuable perspective on the consequences of what
we eat by comparing our diet to those of hunter-gatherers who
survive into the present time. Among the Bushmen of Botswana,
in the Kalahari desert of southern Africa, for example, diseases of
modern civilization such as cancer[8] and cardiovascular disease are
practically unknown. The Bushmen consume a variety of coarse
vegetables and rather tough, low-fat animal meat in an amount that
coincides with their caloric needs. Consequently, although their
weight can vary by a few pounds, Bushmen stay lean throughout
their entire lives. Their only sweets are a local berry that has to be
picked laboriously from a thorny bush, and a few compact-sized
wild fruits that would fail to satisfy an American sweet tooth
accustomed to Famous Amos chocolate chip cookies, iced
Dunkin' Donuts, and Ben and Jerry's ice cream. For all their
seeming deprivation, however, the Bushmen's aerobic fitness—
gauged by measuring the maximum intake of oxygen from a breath
of air—is about a third higher than in American men of the same
age. And their strength and endurance, though not comparable to
Olympic-quality athletes, are markedly superior to the U.S.
average.

The diets of the Bushmen and similar primitive societies have
been analyzed by S. Boyd Eaton and Melvin J. Konner of Emory
University, who strongly suggest that by emulating preurban societies we can prevent diet-related diseases of civilization.[9] According to their study, released in 1985, the fat intake of these
primitive peoples is about 20 percent of total calories, or half the
current intake in the United States. The ratio of unsaturated to
saturated fats is appreciably higher, as is their intake of fiber: about
forty-five grams per day compared to a puny fifteen grams or less
in the United States. Their intake of vitamin C—from fresh fruits
and vegetables—is four times the U.S. level. Their consumption
of refined carbohydrates is virtually nil.

Such diets have sustained cultures for centuries and are appropriate to the nutritional and energy needs of the societies that developed them. When circumstances change, the natural controls vanish and the diet becomes skewed. It has happened often, and always with the introduction of refined sugar.

2

The Fat of the Land

"Gluttony is not a secret vice."
—Orson Welles

TO JUDGE from the jogging stampede of the 1970s and 1980s, and the phenomenal growth of diet and fitness industries, we've finally gotten the message and are slimming down and shaping up with a vengeance. On hand to reassure us like Stepford High cheerleaders are sleek and trim physical ideals pitching low-calorie processed delights on television and in magazines. If all the hoopla is to be believed, we must be the most physically fit generation of Americans ever.

But before giving ourselves a pat on the back, let's take a look at the facts.

We Americans are actually getting fatter, and have been for the last thirty years. Rather than shaping up, we are slipping back. A recent survey conducted at the University of Michigan reveals that those who have gained the most pounds are those who have tried hardest to lose them.[1] These are women aged twenty-five to thirty-four—the same age group that keeps the diet industry in business. Not only have these young women put on extra flab over the years, but there are significantly more of them who are obese than in other age groups.

"From 1960 to 1980," pointed out Dr. J. Richard Landis, one of the study's principal researchers, "the percentage of white women aged twenty-five to thirty-four who were obese increased from 13.3 percent to 17.1 percent of the population. The percentage of obese black women increased from 28.8 percent to 31 percent."[2]

Men of all age groups also gained weight, the study showed, but not enough to indicate a steep upward trend. This doesn't let men off the hook, however. According to the actuarial studies of insurance companies, the majority of American men were already overweight prior to the University of Michigan study.[3] Another survey, conducted by the National Center for Health Statistics, showed that the American male, on average, had gained four pounds from 1962 to 1972.

An increase in height may seem to account for our weight gain, but the canny statisticians have taken this into account.[4] Current estimates are that the typical American female is from fifteen to thirty pounds overweight, and her male counterpart is from twenty to thirty pounds overweight.

What is equally surprising is the fact that although we are gaining weight, we are actually eating less and getting fewer calories than our grandparents and great-grandparents did seventy-five years ago.

The obvious explanation for this apparent contradiction is our increasingly sedentary life-style. Since World War II automation and mechanization has largely replaced the labor formerly performed by farmers and factory workers. The majority of Americans now work in service jobs where physical exertion is practically nonexistent. Our reliance on the automobile has further reduced our energy turnover, and television makes us all immobile observers.

By the mid-1970s, many Americans were feeling this unprecedented decline in physical activity where it shows—in the waistline. To compensate, millions of Americans attempted to eat less by going on diets and buying scores of weight-reducing products that had flooded the market. Others more successfully fought the battle of the bulge by turning play into work. Jogging, running, aerobics, and similar energy-burning recreations indicated a spontaneous reaction to our involuntarily enforced inactivity. A 1977 Gallup Poll found that nearly 47 percent of Americans were exercising regularly, or about twice the percentage of 1961. To George Gallup, this was "one of the most dramatic changes in American life-styles to have taken place in recent decades."

On the face of it, dieting and exercising would seem to be the only means at hand to control our runaway weight gain. Neither, however, gets to the heart of the dilemma. Unless we rethink our sweet and sticky all-American diet, we usually fail on both counts.

Ask yourself: If dieting really worked, would there be such an endless variety of "Seven-Day Miracle," "Low Carbo-Cal," "High-Protein," "Grapefruit," "Fat-Free," "Famous Spa Plan," and you-name-it diets? The majority of these commercialized regimens are crash, or semi-starvation, diets. Yes, you will lose weight at first, but the body will adjust by lowering its metabolism. As a result, you will require fewer calories than before to maintain your weight.

When you go on a stringent diet your natural body instincts come into play, triggering a starvation response. Your body has no idea that it is you who is denying it food. Rather, it reacts as it did aeons ago when game was scarce or in times of famine. To retain its remaining calories, until the emergency is over, it slows down the metabolism rate and burns fat reserves progressively slower. In some people, particularly the obese, the metabolism rate cools down by as much as 15 percent. This is why, after the first two weeks or so, many dieters find it virtually impossible to shed more pounds.[5]

By then, most dieters are so frustrated and hungry that they rush

back to the refrigerator and cookie jar. Those most likely to be
foiled by the starvation response are dieters who were fat children.
These individuals have developed abnormally large fat cells that
persist throughout life. No matter how hard they try to slim down,
their fat cells are constantly crying out to be fed.

Because the previous regimen failed to work, dieters usually go
on to another plan, and then another. And the end result is not
weight loss but weight gain. In a much-quoted study by Dr.
Richard Keesey at the University of Wisconsin,[6] laboratory rats
were reduced in weight by 19 percent, and then fed a rich diet. At
the end of a week their weight was compared to rats which had not
slimmed down but had eaten the same food. The deprived rats
gained twice as much weight as they had previously lost. The
control group showed only a small weight gain. What had happened was that enforced starvation had prompted the animals'
survival instincts to store more calories than they had previously.
This "rebound" factor is why dieters end up with an increased
appetite and more pounds than they had before. Meanwhile, the
body is still on guard, burning fat slowly until it seems safe to return
to the normal metabolic rate. All the while, fat keeps accumulating.

All metabolisms are not created equal, however. Dr. Albert B.
Lowenfels of New York Medical College in Valhalla, New York,
suggests that those of northern European stock and American
Indians adapted to their harsh climates by evolving a "thrifty
gene" that stores fat with super efficiency. The ancestors of these
people probably lived close to glaciers during the last Ice Age. The
gene is still in place and may be responsible for their high cholesterol rates and frequent gallbladder disorders. Swedish women,
Dr. Lowenfels pointed out, have gallstone frequency rates of 22
percent. By contrast, African and Greek women, who live in warm
climates, have rates of about 2 percent.[7]

Another self-delusion shared by millions of weight-conscious

Americans is the belief that no-calorie sweeteners will reduce weight while satisfying taste buds. The American Cancer Society dismissed this myth in a 1986 survey which showed that of 78,000 women interviewed, those who had gained the most weight were the heaviest users of artificial sweeteners. Another study, conducted by J.E. Blundell, a psychologist at Leeds University in England, showed that people who drank water sweetened with aspartame felt hungrier an hour later than those who drank plain water.[8]

These and other investigations suggest that the more convincingly artificial sweeteners taste like sugar, the more effectively they stimulate the appetite. The history of artificial sweeteners indicates they may well initiate cravings for the real thing. Since 1975 our consumption of artificial sweeteners tripled, while our use of sugar rose annually by about one pound per person. Because sugar makes up about 22 percent of per capita calories, much of it hidden in processed and fast foods, replacing it with artificial sweeteners would probably not help much. Researchers theorize that substituting artificial sweeteners for half the sugar we eat would only cut total calories by about 5 percent.

Even without sugar, artificially sweetened cookies, cakes, and ice cream still contain substantial amounts of butter or other fats, which are even more pounds-inducing than sugar. Fat has nine calories per gram, versus sugar's four calories. Sweet 'n Low, NutraSweet, and Sweet One may signal the body to produce insulin to stabilize blood sugar levels, producing hunger, fatigue, irritability, and other symptoms of low-level hypoglycemia (see Chapter 6). At any rate, no matter which sweetener you choose, you are merely substituting one poison for another.

What all sweeteners and fats have in common is an involuntary raising of the body's "setpoint." A kind of internal thermostat, the setpoint determines the natural balance between your fat and muscle. Individual settings vary—some are low, some are high— but all control the body's nutritional equilibrium. Dieting, then, is in effect an attack on one's natural setpoint. By calling into play our starvation response we crank up our "appestats" to eat more food, even though the body doesn't need it. In a healthy individual who eats a balanced diet, the brain's setpoint device keeps body weight at a fairly constant level. A well-functioning setpoint will accommodate minor dietary lapses or emotional ups and downs, and the individual's weight will vary by no more than four or five pounds, which has no effect on health. It's that extra twenty, thirty, or forty pounds that poses well-documented dangers.

Diet pills, called "appetite suppressants" in the trade, also wreak havoc with the setpoint. These lower the setpoint, and the individual loses weight, but only as long as the dosage continues. The appestat adjusts to its lowered, drug-induced caloric require-ments. When the dosage is stopped, weight ultimately shoots back to its former level—and beyond. To maintain a weight loss with diet pills would mean using them throughout your lifetime, not a very desirable prospect for someone who is probably already addicted to sugar and other dangerous substances.

Smoking offers another unhealthy way to lower the setpoint and raise the metabolism. On average, cigarette smokers are trimmer than nonsmokers even though they may eat as many as 250 more calories daily.[9] Years ago, tobacco manufacturers pitched cigarettes to the public as a diet aid. But cigarettes, like diet pills, seem to stimulate rather than suppress appetite. What happens next is that the nicotine in cigarettes turns down the setpoint and thus prevents weight gain. Conversely, when smokers give up the habit, the setpoint is raised and the individual gains weight.

One of the most effective ways of taking off weight, as our fitness mavens have learned, is exercise. Even as little as a half hour each day will lower the setpoint and recharge the metabolism for several hours afterward. The more vigorous your program and the further you jog or run, of course, the most lasting the effect. Dieting, which requires no physical effort at all, may seem the easier solution to sedentary fatties, but it is the burning of calories that makes the difference. Research has shown that those in the least-active professions—lawyers, accountants, managers, and clerks—are heavier than outdoor workers, mechanics, postmen and professional athletes. And when did you last see an Olympic runner carrying extra weight?

But exercise is only part of the solution. Being overweight or obese are not diseases in themselves; they are warning signs of nutritional disaster. They are a symptom of a diet high in calories but incomplete in other essential nutrients. And ''yo-yo'' dieting virtually eliminates nutrients that are already lacking. The brain must have a steady and complete supply of these nutrients to maintain the body's chemical equilibrium. A lifetime diet of sweets, white bread, pastries, sugared cereals, soft drinks, and fast foods serves only to distort the brain's capacity to control appetite and metabolism and to prevent illness. Inevitably, a reducing diet is sought to eliminate only the visible signs of an individual's problem.

Over the years, the body has gotten used to a daily intake of quickly absorbed refined carbohydrates, and it has tried to deal as best it could with these demands. Couple increased sugar sensitivity with the added problems of alcohol, stress, and drugs, by prescription or otherwise, and you have a profoundly abused biochemistry. Many overweight people show an abnormal sugar tolerance and have elevated blood levels of cholesterol and free fatty acids.

Eating less and exercising more will work only briefly unless you reset your setpoint by eliminating refined, simple carbohydrates from your daily diet. Since they provide substantial bulk, and thereby limit the amount your stomach can hold, you can eat as many whole grains, such as wild rice, wheat berries, bulgur wheat, buckwheat, and brown rice, as you can hold. By eating whole grains, vegetables, and fruits, you will consume only a fraction of the calories you formerly obtained from refined sugar and starches (which are converted into sugar in the stomach).

In his highly readable book *Fit or Fat?* Covert Bailey maintains that the best method of retooling one's internal chemistry is a regular schedule of aerobic exercises. These increase the heart rate and bring oxygen to the muscles, where a significant amount of fat is stored. In an average person, the muscles contain from 12 percent to 22 percent fat; in professional athletes the percentage is only a third as much. In the overweight and the obese, the percentage is much higher. When the body is subjected to a faulty diet of sugar and starch, fats, and/or alcohol, and there is no opportunity to exercise, fat is substituted for some of the muscle tissue.[10]

By reducing your body's capacity for energy storage, you will be reducing your chance of a premature death from diabetes, high blood pressure, heart attacks, cancer, and kidney disorders. You will also get rid of the added burden on your musculoskeletal frame, which can result in arthritis, back disorders, and gout, all common complaints of the obese and overweight.

3

The Candy-Coated Teat

"How do you judge the infant's diet if not in terms of the entire life history?"

—*Carlton Fredericks*

OFFER AN INFANT a bottle filled with tomato juice and it will wrinkle its already wrinkled little brow in angry rejection of the sour taste. Offer it a bottle filled with milk laced with sugar and it will suck avidly at the nipple. The baby is not being self-indulgent but merely exhibiting a built-in taste for mother's milk, which it needs to survive and grow.

In her infinite wisdom Mother Nature has endowed us all with an innate preference for the sweet and the fat, which we manifest from the very beginning of life. In evolutionary terms human beings like sweet foods because we learned aeons ago, by trial and error, that generally in nature nothing that tastes sweet can make us ill or kill us. Bitter or sour items have the potential to harm us, and a bite of an unknown fruit or vegetable can indicate whether it is safe (sweet) enough—and ripe enough—to eat.

We like fat foods because, like sweets, they are highly concentrated sources of energy and, in nature, chock-full of vitamins, minerals, and essential fatty acids. In the past foods containing sugar and fat were always in short supply, so our ancestors loaded up on them whenever they could. Experience told them to stock up for a rainy day because a shortage would soon take care of their fat

33

reserves, which rarely, if ever, were given the opportunity to get out of hand.

Our egregious taste for fats and sweets, then, is a product of natural selection built into the taste centers of our brains. This in part helps explain why so many of us develop a can't-say-no addiction to sweet, gooey foods. But it is only part of the story. Behavior counts as much as biology, and a primary reason we get hooked is because of the misguided intentions of parents. For the sake of convenience, and in the name of love, they have become pushers of nutritional junk by giving their kids what they think they want.

When a baby cries often, for example, a syrup-coated pacifier is shoved into its mouth. At three or four months, the infant is given some processed solid baby food. Although these are no longer doctored with salt and sugar (except for some strained fruits and puddings) they *did* contain these unnecessary chemicals when most of the readers of this book were babies. (The industry has since tried to compensate by using only the ripest and most sugar-rich ingredients and by adding more of a thickening agent called modified food starch.) From baby food the child progresses to sweetened breakfast cereals, with candy and cake frequently introduced as a reward for good behavior.

The fat baby everybody loved and thought so healthy and cute grows up to be an adult who can't live without hefty doses of sugar and fats in his or her daily fare. The result is a permanent weight problem that sets the stage for debilitating illness in later life. Given a proper diet rich in natural, unadulterated complex carbohydrates, lean proteins, and a minimum of fats, a normal child would have grown out of his sweet tooth after adolescence, when the body adjusts to the lesser caloric demands of maturity. And we wonder why 12 percent of elementary-schoolers and 20 percent to 30 percent of high school teenagers are overweight.[1]

Posters from the U.S. Department of Agriculture urging children to choose balanced meals from the Four Basic Food Groups adorn school walls everywhere, but the dream falls far short of reality. In a U.S. government survey taken between 1976 and 1980, it was found that kids aged one to five drank as much Kool-Aid and carbonated colas as they did orange juice. Children aged six to eleven were more likely to choose cookies over apples, oranges, and bananas as a snack food. And twelve- to seventeen-year-olds regarded potato chips and corn chips as their vegetable of choice—over salad and such apparently bygone staples as carrots and peas.[2]

These shocking findings, gathered by the National Health and Nutrition Examination Survey (HANES), are the most recent figures available but sales figures indicate they still hold true. HANES figures show that our children grow up on soft drinks, cookies, brownies, ice cream, Twinkies, Fritos, Slurpees, Popsicles, hot dogs, Big Macs, white bread, and bologna—in other words, a diet of sugar, fat, salt, and more fat, salt, and sugar. At the bottom of the list of childhood food preferences are fresh fruit, cabbage, green beans, tomatoes, chicken, and lean beef. Fish barely makes the chart.

Today, children's eating habits are likely to be shaped not only by their parents but by television commercials cleverly slanted to make junk foods irresistibly appealing. It's difficult for a parent to compete with operations like Mars candy, which spends $140 million a year on advertising, and Nabisco cookies, which spends $38 million, and Coca-Cola, which spends $152 million.[3] They each have their eye on the $4.6 billion in allowance money that Children's Market Research Inc. of New York estimates that thirty million children between ages six and fourteen have at their disposal. And that's not to mention the $40 to $50 billion in annual family spending that CMR believes kids influence.

Parents protest from time to time but the come-ons continue to air, turning our children into flaccid couch potatoes whose only exercise comes from reaching into snack food bags. These unhealthy products have become so much a part of their brief life experience that children even crave them as toys. A recent visit to a Toys "Я" Us outlet in New Jersey revealed an entire aisle devoted to what the chain calls "playfoods." There were plastic Dunkin' Donuts, appropriately scented synthetically, in vanilla and chocolate, Baskin-Robbins ice cream cones, Kentucky Fried Chicken, Burger King Whoppers—which can be disassembled into bun, cheese, onion, tomato, pickles, lettuce—and, of course, a side of plastic French fries and fried onion rings.

If your child so desires, he or she can now dress the part. Sears reports that its line of McKids clothing, embossed with the familiar golden arch, reached almost $100 million in sales in 1988. Burger King offers a less extensive line of accessories, and, of course, Coca-Cola clothing and luggage has been around for many years.

Take an hour next Saturday and watch some kidvid programs with your child. In one study, a professor of dietetics at the University of Delaware taped all the programs broadcast by the three major networks on Saturday morning. She found that more than three-quarters of the 225 commercials she monitored were for "products of low nutritional value" such as canned Spaghetti-Os, presweetened fruit beverages, soft drinks, and microwaveable imitation milkshakes.[4]

The major networks all abide by the Legal Breakfast Rule, which means only that in a commercial for a sugared breakfast cereal, an adequately nutritious breakfast must be shown. Without skipping a breath, the charged-up announcer will say something along the order of, "Sugarific Cereal can be a part of this wholesome breakfast." The images of a pitcher of milk, a glass of orange juice, hot buttered toast, and some sliced fruit are gone before you've had time to get the point. CBS's Television Network Advertising Guidelines state that these messages must be aired "for at least three seconds."[5]

Television's ambiguous, self-imposed rulings do nothing more than pay lip service to public concerns about the advertising power of the food industry. In fact, these telegraphed messages may actually be giving children the wrong impression by seeming to imply that such-and-such presweetened breakfast cereal is necessary for a balanced breakfast. The good and the bad are likely to be confused in the mind of a six-year-old who watches a lot of Saturday morning television. Anyone who has ever seen a child throwing a tantrum in a supermarket until mom fills the cart with sweetened nothings seen on television knows the effects of this kind of conditioning.

While television remains the most insidious influence on children's taste buds, advertisers have launched new lines of attack to pull dollars from parental pockets, this time in print. Not long ago, the popular *Archie* comics produced a special issue, sponsored by General Foods Corporation; its featured character was a pitcher of Kool-Aid. And every four months *McCall's* magazine was inserting into its five million copies a smaller-sized magazine for juveniles called *Betsy McCall*. And another million copies of *Betsy* went to every K-Mart store, where they were distributed free to their intended audience: girls from six to twelve years of age. *Betsy* appeared to be a real magazine, but upon closer look it was apparent that not all was what it seemed to be. Recipes called for such ingredients as Pepsi Cola and Mott's puddings, products that turned out to have ads on nearby pages. "The magazine is clearly an advertorial," said a spokesman for *McCall's*, when the magazine was accused of not clearly labeling *Betsy* as such. "It's a product of the advertising department. It's all paid for."

The question remains, can a young girl reading *Betsy* tell the difference between what's an ad and what's not? Studies have shown that children watching television often cannot tell the difference, because commercials are made to be as entertaining as the programs they sponsor.[6] There were a lot of processed food coupons in *Betsy,* but the magazine's most alarming features were the fun-laden, page-length games that were nothing more than product promotions. In General Foods' ''Pebble Bedrock Races,'' for instance, players were instructed to find the buried treasure of ''yabba dabba delicious Post Fruity Pebbles and Cocoa Pebbles cereal.'' Both breakfast foods, if you can call them that, have been roundly condemned by nutritionists everywhere because they are just about the sweetest cereals on the market. They contain more than half their weight in sugar.[7]

Heredity, environment, and nutrition are the major determinants of a child's potential in later life, and of these nutrition is the single most important factor. It is also the most controllable factor. Children need extra calories to supply the chemicals that form growing tissues, especially the muscles, bones, blood, and teeth. Extra calories are also needed for repairing damage caused by illnesses and injuries. But the calories they require are not the empty calories of refined sugar and processed starches. In replacing protein, vitamins, minerals, and fiber with an excess of simple carbohydrates, saturated fats, and artificial ingredients, many children are eating their way to obesity and assorted health problems that will manifest themselves in later life.

Unwittingly, many mothers reinforce their child's natural preference for sweet foods. When a child refuses a bitter or sourish vegetable, for instance, mom will probably sweeten the spinach or broccoli with sugar or throw it down the garbage disposal and never serve it again. And if the child does manage to eat the proffered vegetable, mom provides a sweet or a dessert as a reward. This reinforces the child's belief—learned from television—that sweet, empty-calorie food is superior to good nourishing food. By the time the child reaches adolescence, a period of rapid development in which the need for body-building food increases, it may be too late to reeducate the taste buds.

The schoolroom, with its captive audience, would seem to be an ideal arena for nutritionists who bemoan the dietary habits of America's children and want to integrate healthy habits into their lives. But so far, few schools have comprehensive and compulsory health education programs. In a 1988 survey conducted by the Metropolitan Life Foundation and Louis Harris & Associates, it was estimated that about eight million public school students get no significant health education. The survey, which polled 4,738 students in 199 schools, revealed that less than 22 percent gave much consideration to the nutritional quality of the foods they buy. Nineteen percent usually skipped breakfast on schooldays, and 13 percent got no exercise at all.

Ask parents what their child is being taught in school about food, and you will probably get a surprised look. Most parents just don't know. Of the 500 parents questioned in the survey, only one in ten had made inquiries about health education of school officials or had consulted with other parents.

Of the schools that do have health and nutrition programs, educators report that pupils quickly pick up the message and buy fewer candies, cookies, cakes, sodas, chewing gum, and the like.[8] An exemplary program is Growing Healthy, developed by the National Center for Health Education in New York City and funded by the Federal Centers for Disease Control. Learning is made into a multimedia experience that lingers in a child's mind as effectively as a television commercial. The human body is diagrammed on the floor and students walk through the various organs to experience vicariously the effects of such bad habits as smoking, taking drugs, and eating the wrong foods.

"It's hard for a child—anyone, for that matter—to understand that what tastes good is not necessarily good for you," points out Vicki Lansky in her book, *The Taming of the C.A.N.D.Y. Monster*. Lansky defines C.A.N.D.Y. as Continuously Advertised Nutritionally Deficient Yummies, and advises parents not to have sweets in the house. "Tell your children that the reason you don't want them to eat these extraneous foods is BECAUSE YOU LOVE THEM and you want them to be strong and healthy."

Adolescence is the last chance parents have to wean their offspring from the sugared nipple. Food habits acquired during this period usually endure throughout life. Teenagers are a contrary lot, however, and by then they may be too overweight and passive to want to make the effort. If sweets are restricted from the beginning, most teenagers will grow out of their sweet tooth after adolescence when extra calories are no longer needed.

4

Sugar: An Unnatural History

"Sugar-plummes heateth the blood. . . . Rotteth the teeth . . . and withall, causeth many times a loathsome stinking breath."

Klinike on the Diet of Disease
—Dr. James Hurt
(1633)

No ONE KNEW what to make of sugar when it arrived in Western Europe in the dusty saddlebags of Arab traders during the eighth century. To the royal minority who could afford the stuff, sugar was an exotic seasoning from the Orient to be used sparingly as a food accent and as a medicine. Called "stone honey" because it was sweet and pressed into oblong cakes, sugar was too costly to be used for anything else. To the commonfolk, sugar was so out of reach it might as well not have existed. Transforming the dangerous white granules into a luxury affordable for all would require centuries of geopolitical struggle and human misery.

By necessity, if you had the wherewithal or were lucky enough to find some in the wild, the sweetener of choice was honey. Ordinary sweet tooths had to wait until summer, when apples, melons, berries, and other fruits came into season. Those blessed with a bountiful crop could preserve the surplus by setting it out to dry in the sun so that the fruit could be enjoyed in winter. Sun-drying retained many of fruits' original vitamins, minerals, and

41

enzymes, and in the process greatly increased their sugar content. Fresh apricots, for instance, have a sugar content of approximately 15 percent, but after evaporation of their moisture, the sugar content goes up to over 70 percent. Sun-dried fruits are still with us (although commercial sulfured brands are to be avoided), and they remain a satisfying natural treat.

Arabs weren't the first to use sugar, they were merely the first ones to push it. Sugarcane had been cultivated in India at least a millenium before the Persians got hold of it. This tall, perennial, tropical plant of the grass family was a familiar sight in India as long ago as 345 B.C., when soldiers of Alexander the Great's army reported finding a "honey-bearing reed" as they explored the Indus Valley. They noted that locals seemed to enjoy chewing on the raw cane and especially liked to drink the juice as a fermented beverage. Indians called the plant *sarkara,* a Sanskrit word from which we derived "sugar," and referred to the unevenly shaped solids that formed when cane juice was boiled as *khanda,* from which we got the word candy.[1]

That mankind has lived most of his existence without refined sugar is apparent when we take a look at the great books. Sugar is not mentioned as such in the Bible, the Talmud, or the Koran, so presumably Adam and Eve got along very well without it in the Garden of Eden. Although references to sweetness abound in the Bible, the sweets are milk and honey, and probably nectar extracted by mashing ripe fruits.

That isn't to say that sugar was unknown in the ancient West. The Romans called it "Indian salt," and Dioscorides, a writer of Nero's time, gave it its Latin name: *saccharum.* Dioscorides described sugar as a "sort of concreted honey which is saccharum found in canes in India and Arabia Felix; it is in consistence like salt and brittle between the teeth."

The Romans, like the Europeans who later rediscovered it,

considered sugar primarily to be a medicine. Mystical healing qualities were attributed to the white crystals, which were offered as a cure for everything from dyspepsia, boils, wounds, impotence, and hair loss. Perhaps medicine was what refined sugar was really meant to be. Clinicians have demonstrated that when mixed with a salve, table sugar can speed up the healing of some wounds and burns. And a mixture of glucose and saltwater taken intravenously has saved many a victim of severe diarrhea.[2]

The Arabs preferred to eat their sugar, and once started they couldn't seem to get enough of it. But even before they happened upon sugarcane, which they no doubt considered a lucky break, Arabs had been eating sweets for centuries. Still a favorite in the Middle East is juice pressed from very ripe dates, which is allowed to evaporate into a thick syrup. This viscous, highly flavored, and relatively nutritious sweetener was used for puddings and to make alcoholic drinks. Date trees were—and still are—tapped for their sugary sap, in the same way American Indians on the other side of the world tapped maple trees.

From the eleventh to the fourteenth centuries, bands of civilians and soldiers straggled across Europe to tame the heathen Arabs and reclaim the Holy Land in nine so-called People's Crusades. The infidels didn't quite succeed but they did develop a taste for sugar, which the more enterprising feudal lords brought home to cultivate in North Africa. Considering how much sugar Europeans were ultimately to consume, the Arabs may have been the victors after all. Revenge, as they say, is sweet.

There never was enough honey to go around, and by the fifteenth century there was even less available. Oil lamps were replacing beeswax candles, so fewer monasteries, the main commercial source of honey, were keeping bees. Europe's shortage of sweeteners didn't last long, however, and soon plantations in the

New World were providing sugar cheaply and in unlimited quantities.[3]

The introduction of coffee from Arabia increased sugar demand markedly, to feed the sugar hunger of thousands of Europeans who regularly visited the local café or *kaffehaus*. Among the continent's most avid coffee fanciers were the Dutch, whose brisk trade with the American colonies and the East Indies brought them a new affluence.[4] One of their favored imports was sugar, which had previously been a luxury. Their demand for sugar was so excessive that by 1660, Amsterdam boasted more than fifty sugar refineries and had become the carbohydrate capital of Europe.

Among the legacies the Dutch have left behind are the works of Rembrandt and other master painters—and depictions of the disastrous effects of sugar on the teeth. You can see examples of both great craftsmanship and great sugar damage in any major art museum. In 1989 two Boston dentists, Harvey and Sheldon Peck, examined a number of canvases by Rembrandt and other artists of the period and came to the conclusion that many of the Dutchmen depicted were "dental cripples." Writing in the trade journal *Dental Abstracts,* the Peck brothers determined that many sixteenth-century Dutch were "endentulous"—toothless—and that others showed signs of tooth decay. Toothbrushes to scrub away bacteria that thrive on sugar were as yet unheard of, and the only dental hygiene was "the occasional postprandial toothpick."[5]

One of the few voices of reason at the time was the baritone of James Hurt. A natural healer whose teachings were considered unorthodox, Hurt was an early proponent of preventing illness with diet and a wholesome life-style. Hurt preferred to write his self-help books in English, the language of the commonfolk, rather than Latin, the language of scholars, which meant he was shunned by the Royal Society, the American Medical Association of his day. Dr. Hurt knew what he was talking about, however, and his comments on sugar in *Klinike on the Diet of Disease,* published in 1633, still hold true:

> Sugar in itself be opening and cleansing, yet being much used produceth dangerous effects on the body: as namely, immoderate use thereof, as also of sweet confections, and Sugar-plummes heateth the blood, ingendreth obstructions, cachexias, consumptions, rotteth the teeth, making them look blacke; and withal causeth many times a loathsome stinking breath. And therefore let young people especially beware how they meddle too much with it.

What had made so much sugar available in so short a time was slave labor. Spain, a leader in the sugar trade, pressed natives into service when it set up plantations in Cuba and the Greater Antilles Islands, but there were too few natives to harvest and process the cane. The Spanish solution was to buy black workers in Africa in the belief that only Africans could work in the brutal heat of the summer tropics. The English, Dutch, French, and other European countries soon followed suit, and the Caribbean and South American wilderness was dotted with plantations worked by black slaves. Competition between exploitive European nations ensured that there would be plenty of sugar for all.

Meanwhile, new uses were being found for sugar. Jam made its debut in the early 1700s, and *koekjes,* small cakes the English called cookies, appeared in Dutch bakeshops. Master chefs mixed sugar with ground cocoa beans and created a myriad of new sweets: hot chocolate, chocolate candy, and chocolate cake. Sugar had become so valuable that in 1667 the Dutch were persuaded to hand New York over to England to get back its plantations in captured Suriname.

Sugar was slow to take hold in the United States, however, since few colonists could afford to buy it. Most Americans, like their Puritan forebears, were frugal and believed that sweets and other luxury foods were to be eaten only occasionally and as a treat or a reward. The Puritans, of course, ate no refined sugar at all, which no doubt helped account for their incredible stamina. America's taste for sugar increased with the introduction of processed foods following the Civil War, then seemed to wane when sugar shortages during World War I temporarily released them from the growing habit.

But affluence always seems to encourage a taste for sweetness, and during the boom years of the 1920s Americans began to indulge themselves as never before. Previously, table sugar was sold loose by the pound, but now it could be purchased in neat bags and boxes that made it easier to buy and store in home pantries. That the new packaging also jacked up the price didn't seem to matter to most consumers, who showed they preferred convenience over expense. Packaging also greatly increased sales of ice cream by turning it into a portable food that could be carried in a cone or on a stick. Candy, previously available only in boxes and bags by the pound or a fraction thereof, was packaged in small units and given appealing, memorable names. Candy bars were mass-merchandised in grocery stores, drugstores, newsstands, tobacco stores, and other locations with a busy traffic flow. These products eventually became so familiar that brand names like Baby Ruth, Oh Henry!, and Mars are now part of America's popular culture.[6] Similarly, such snack foods as potato chips and cookies were sealed into packages, launching a procession of junk foods that continues to this day.

We can thank the Coca-Cola Company for permanently hooking America and much of the rest of the world on sugared soft drinks. Coca-Cola takes its name from its original ingredients—coca leaves and cola nuts—first blended together in 1886 by Atlanta pharmacist John S. Pemberton as a cure for headaches and hangovers. Pemberton eventually sold the business to another druggist, Asa G. Candler, who inaugurated an advertising policy that has continued to this day. The Coca-Cola Company has spent more money on advertising for its product than any other company in Madison Avenue history.

Around the turn of the century, Coca-Cola expanded its already growing market by taking the syrup out of local soda fountains and premixing it with soda water in bottles. To its growing number of fanciers, the beverage was called simply "Coke," an appellation shunned by the company because it was (and is) a popular nickname for cocaine, which was part of the original formula. An early Coca-Cola advertisement made reference to the beverage's stimulative effects, calling it the "ideal brain tonic" and claiming it was a delightful way to "relieve exhaustion." The traces of cocaine that remained in the company's still-secret formula were ultimately removed, and today it is the sugar and the caffeine that make Coke so addictive.

An attempt to reformulate the soft drink in the 1980s was met with such a public outrage that the company was forced to return to its old formula—although not quite. Classic Coke does not taste the same as its forebear because the company has switched to cheaper high fructose corn syrup.

Coke, like the various sugars that have sustained it, has reached across the oceans into nearly every country of the world, and to millions of people it remains a symbol of the United States.

Most of the sugar Americans consume is grown here at home and comes from sugar beets, which produce a product identical to cane's. We can thank Napoleon Bonaparte, no slouch when it came to sweets, for developing the sugar beet after the Napoleonic wars cut off French sugar supplies in the Caribbean.

Refining sugar, especially cane, is a demanding, arduous process. The harvested cane is first chopped into small pieces, then
crushed by huge rollers. Water is added and the juice squeezed out,
filtered, and poured into heating vats. Powdered lime is added to
separate out most of the extraneous matter. The heated brown
liquid begins to clarify as the unwanted materials settle to the
bottom of the tank. Boiling continues until the moisture is released
and the liquid reduces into a thick, viscous mash. This is pumped
into vacuum pots to further concentrate the juice. Nearly dry, the
crystals go into a centrifuge to spin off the molasses. Again heated
to the boiling point, the reliquefied sugar is passed repeatedly
through charcoal filters. For additional whitening, ash from burned
beef bones is used. Finally, the sugar is condensed into crystals.
The resulting product is as pure a chemical as anything you might
find in a chemist's laboratory.[7]

Removed in the refining process are about sixty-four food elements. A, D, and the B complex vitamins are destroyed, and the
minerals calcium, manganese, iron, phosphorus, and other trace
elements are leached into the residue, along with all the fiber,
amino acids, enzymes, and unsaturated fat. You can get back some
of the B vitamins in a by-product called blackstrap molasses, but
the remainder is in the solids, which are processed as livestock
food.

Chemical fertilizers and herbicides are used in cultivation,
which is another reason not to eat it.

Today's sugar trade is an international megabusiness that moves
and shakes a number of Caribbean Basin, South American and
Pacific republics. The largest producers of cane sugar are Brazil,
Cuba, and Australia, while the United States, France, and Russia
lead in beet production. The U.S. still doesn't make enough sugar
to satisfy demand, however, and we have to import 750,000 tons
more, mostly from Caribbean countries.

U.S. sugar law, in force since 1982, sets the American price at triple the world market price, to protect American sugar producers. This has had the effect of increasing the popularity of corn sweeteners and pushing some American food processors over the border to Canada, where they can prefabricate cookies, candies, and cake mixes with cheaper sugar. The economy of the Philippines depends on America's sweet tooth to keep it going, so Congress voted, in 1987, to import an extra 300,000 tons of their raw materials. Part of the deal was that the refined product would be reexported at the lower world price, with the government making up the difference out of our pockets by giving American refiners surplus commodities.[8] It's an old story: the consumer being ripped off by sugar.

THE MANY FACES OF SUGAR

In addition to familiar white refined table sugar, food processors have at their command a variety of other sugars, as follows. Nutritionally, the only real advantage of one over another is sweetness and a tiny savings in calories. Fructose, for example, is about 70 percent sweeter than table sugar, or sucrose, which means that a lesser amount can achieve the same degree of sweetness. Maltose, on the other hand, is only about two-thirds as sweet as sucrose and requires a greater amount to match its sweetness. All sugars contain about four calories per gram.

Sucrose: White granulated sugar, commonly used in the home, refined from sugarcane and sugar beets. It is a nearly pure chemical and will keep indefinitely. The "fine" grade is what we use at the table. "Ultrafine" and "very fine" are used in commercial baked products, cake mixes, soft drinks, and candy coatings because they mix well with other finely divided ingredients.

Turbinado sugar: Partially refined sucrose. It is often mistakenly referred to as raw sugar.

Brown sugar: Sucrose colored with a molasses-flavored syrup. Valued for flavor and color, brown sugar is often added to baked beans, gingerbread, and meat sauces and glazes.

Dextrose: The commercial name for glucose, or blood sugar. Also called corn sugar, dextrose is about half as sweet as sucrose. All sugars are ultimately converted to glucose by the body.

Invert sugar: The end product of heating a solution of sucrose with an acid or enzymes. The process breaks up sucrose into its two components, fructose and glucose, and increases the volume of the sucrose by about 5 percent. Invert sugar is a syrup that retains moisture and prolongs the freshness of baked goods. Because it resists crystallization, it is often used instead of sugar in soft drinks, jams and jellies, candy bars, and canned fruit.

Fructose: Fruit sugar, a component of invert sugar, usually obtained from corn. Also called levulose, fructose is intensely sweet and highly soluble and, until recently, was reserved for vitamin pills and bitter-tasting medications such as cough syrups. It has lately turned up in so-called diet products with the false claim that it is intrinsically more healthful than ordinary sugar.

Lactose: Milk sugar, present in the milk of every mammal. Usually extracted from whey and skim milk, lactose is not very sweet and not very soluble. It is used primarily to add bulk to pharmaceuticals and in some baked goods and infant formulas.

Maltose: Also called malt sugar, formed by the action of yeast on starch. Much less sweet than sucrose, maltose is usually combined with dextrose in breads and sweet rolls.

Corn syrup: A viscous liquid obtained by heating cornstarch in the presence of enzymes, a process that converts the cornstarch into a multiple sugar containing maltose, dextrose, glucose, and other polysaccharides. Because corn syrup has a distinct flavor and is much less sweet than sugar, it is generally used in combination with other sweeteners.

High fructose corn syrup: Corn syrup treated with an enzyme that converts some of its glucose to fructose. Known in the trade as HFCS, this relatively new sweetener has largely replaced corn syrup as a food additive. HFCS is cheaper than sugar and nearly as sweet, and has the added advantage of lengthening the shelf life of products because of its moisture-retaining properties. Look for it in candies, tomato sauces, condiments, canned fruits, and baked goods.

Honey: Essentially an invert sugar containing sucrose, glucose, fructose, and other sugars and water. Once touted as a nutritional supplement, honey actually has such minute trace amounts of minerals as to be insignificant to human needs. Although some honeys are even sweeter than fructose, others are less sweet than sucrose and add rather than subtract calories.

Molasses: The juice extracted from sugarcane or sugar beets after the sucrose has been removed in the refining process. This sticky brown liquid retains some of the nutrients that occur naturally in the plants as well as some sugar. Because it has a strong taste and is somewhat bitter, molasses is infrequently added to prepared foods. It is the closest any commercial sweetener comes to a whole food, however, since it retains iron, calcium, and some B vitamins, although in unreliable amounts.

5

Me, a Sugarholic?

*"[O]ur three basic needs, for food, security and love,
are so intertwined that we cannot straightly think of one
without the other."*

—*M.F.K. Fisher*

- Do you habitually face the day with a doughnut, coffee cake, or a sweetened croissant?
- Do your taste buds require ketchup, mayonnaise, relish, or "special sauce" on nearly everything that can hold it?
- Do you keep sweets in your desk or pocket or purse to give you a needed lift during the day?
- Do you always buy the sweetened variety of frozen or canned fruits, and prefer juice drinks to real juice?
- Do you find yourself making an extra trip to the store when you have run out of soft drinks?
- Do you feel unsatisfied unless you finish a meal with a sweet dessert?
- Do you need a dish of ice cream or a piece of cake before bedtime in order to sleep well?
- Does an eating binge of cookies or candy calm your jangled nerves?

If you answered yes to any of these questions, consider yourself a bona fide sugarholic. Without any conscious intent, you have become addicted to sugar and/or its substitutes.

Like any other addictive substance, sugar creates insatiable cravings that must be satisfied on a regular basis. If you don't get your daily fix, you start to show withdrawal symptoms. These can include weakness and fatigue, headaches, restlessness, anxiety, mental confusion, insomnia, and extreme irritability. Acting like a mood-altering tranquilizer, a cup of sugared coffee, a doughnut, or a chocolate chip cookie will bring you back to normal.[1]

Predictably, as with any addiction, your tolerance level has increased over the years in proportion to the hidden sugars that have been added to America's food supply. Try though you might to abstain from sweets, you find yourself inevitably drawn back to your favorite goodies. No substitute will do. Only sugar will restore your sense of well-being.

If hunger dictated appetite, as with animals in the wild, none of us would have to worry about sugar. But what we eat is influenced in significant ways by the culture we live in. Sugar is not merely a food, it is an American institution. We do more than *consume* sugar, we experience our lives with it. We have even evolved a set of images, dreams, and values based on sugar. For some, it is a term of endearment to call a friend or a spouse "honey" or "sugar." To be wealthy means you are enjoying "the sweet life" and have tasted the "sweet smell of success." And the American popular song *Sugar Time,* a hit of the 1950s, urges us to eat "sugar in the morning, sugar in the evening, sugar at suppertime."

We associate white with purity and goodness, as in the color of a bride's wedding dress or the sterile sheets and scrubbed fixtures of a hospital room. Nothing is whiter than refined white sugar and white flour, of course, and we transfer our emotional feelings to these devalued foodstuffs.[2] Appearance and palatability are too often paramount in our food selections, usually without our being at all aware of it. Advertisers play on our collective psychology, signaling us to buy their "sweet," "crisp," and "moist" products with a body of images and words that appeal to our basic social and cultural values and attitudes.

Every nation has a "food language" that reflects its cultural attitudes toward food. The French are known for their fine wines, the Italians for their pastas, and the Japanese for their raw fish dishes. Americans are known to the world for junk foods that are sugary and synthetic.

Other cultures rely much less on sugar as a food staple than we do. The Japanese, for example, have yet to reach our level of consumption, even though they seem to have acquired a taste for sugar since the introduction of American fast food restaurants. But by and large, the Japanese are not fond of sugary and buttery American sweets, and many respond with nausea at the first bite of such American staples as cheesecake and fudge. To the virgin tongue, American sweets seem to trigger a response similar to the experiences of first-time users of alcohol, tobacco, heroin, morphine, and other addictive drugs.

The biological rewards of eating are obvious: to keep the body functioning and to stay alive. In nature, the body has no trouble balancing the complex mechanism of hunger. When the stomach is no longer filled and when glucose levels in the blood drop, the body tells us it is time to eat. This internal signal, called hunger pangs, is a survival tactic developed by the species through aeons of evolution. When we eat, the body rewards us by ending the hunger pangs and making us feel relaxed and secure.[3]

What can upset this delicate balance is our emotions. When we go on sugar binges, it's probably because our parents taught us to think of sweet foods as a reward or as something to soothe an emotional upset. Eating is a pleasurable activity, of course, and, for a young child, sugar makes it even more pleasurable. This early experience sets the stage for a lifetime of sugar addiction. And as more and more of our food supply becomes processed, manufacturers mask the taste of nutritionally inferior ingredients with tasty and emotionally rewarding sugar. Advertisers help us along with messages that appeal to the child in each of us rather than to our good sense.

Consider the fact that you reinforce your cravings at least three times a day, not including snacks. So, more than a thousand times a year you are being rewarded by your body, society, and yourself. Eating, in this sense, is behavior, and behavior is reinforced by repetition, forming what we call a habit. And unhealthy habits are a major problem in contemporary society.

Another reason many of us turn to food for pleasure rather than for sustenance is anxiety, a generalized feeling of dread that has become commonplace. New research indicates that some Americans become addicts primarily because they are suffering from serious depression or anxiety. In a 1988 study at the New York State Psychiatric Institute, doctors found that many of the alcoholics and drug abusers examined had begun their habit not primarily for "getting high," but because they wanted to "feel better." When treated with imipramine, a drug that blocks depression and anxiety attacks, they were able to cope with their problems and no longer needed alcohol or drugs. These substance abusers, researchers noted, were actually attempting a form of self-medication to relieve the symptoms of their psychological distress.[4]

Sugar can make you feel good too—at least for a couple of hours. Sugar, like all carbohydrates, increases the amount of a brain chemical serotonin. Some of us lack serotonin, which probably works in tandem with our cultural bias toward sugar. But sugar isn't the only source of this chemical. You can also get it from milk, vegetables, and whole grains, but it takes longer to feel the effect. Americans used to the quick fix are not inclined to want to take the time. The only catch with the sugar treatment is that you need to eat a lot of fattening junk all the time.

Sugar is often combined with chocolate—probably America's favorite dessert—which contains a chemical called tyramine, absorbed by the nerves. Tyramine can act as a stimulant or a depressant, which can cause competing reactions with the serotonin in sugar. This head-on collision, researchers say, adds to the addictive quality of chocolate. The five chemicals in chocolate also cause the body to burn sugar faster, urging the chocolate lover to eat more bonbons to satisfy this sugar need. As with any addiction, the chocolate habit can take on a life of its own.

In our Age of Anxiety there are more addictions than ever to choose from, just as there are more people with mental problems. Psychological illness now hospitalizes as many people as physical ailments do. Add to this those in outpatient clinics, in institutions, and who weekly visit private psychiatrists and psychotherapists and you have a total of upward of ten million Americans with mental or emotional problems. This is about three times the number treated for mental illness in 1940.[5]

While these statistics are troubling enough, particularly alarming is the increasing incidence of mental illness among school-age children. About a million and a half of our young people suffer from such serious disorders as depression, psychotic episodes, and schizophrenia. And because many families are too embarrassed to reveal their child's problems, some researchers believe that figure is much larger. Meanwhile, public costs for mental illness have soared to nearly $70 billion and continue to increase.[6]

Social scientists theorize as to why many of today's teenagers become so depressed that they consider taking their own lives. The experts have all failed to come up with an answer, possibly because they are looking in the wrong places.

The most recent study by the Department of Agriculture offers a valuable clue. Although we are eating a few more vegetables and fibrous grains and less saturated fat than we have in the past, we are eating more highly refined, processed carbohydrates than ever before. Only about half of the families surveyed ate foods that meet Recommended Daily Allowances (RDAs) for calcium, vitamin C, vitamin A, some of the B vitamins, and iron. We may live in an age of nutritional awareness, but our diets don't show it. Children, particularly, are gorging on sugar, fats, and salt, and not getting the nutrients essential to physical and mental health.[7]

Adolescents aged from ten to sixteen eat the most nutritionally wanting diets of all age groups according to government statistics. Their food preferences are devastatingly telling. Milk and dairy products have given way to a preference for soft drinks; juices and fruit are being replaced by punches and ades; and a nutritious potato is only acceptable if it is French-fried. Make-at-home meals are less acceptable than processed foods heated in a microwave (the biggest-selling kitchen appliance of the 1980s). Cookies, doughnuts, ice cream, candy, crackers, cupcakes, potato chips, and other eat-and-run items made of sugar, starch, and chemical additives have become the order of the day for too many teenagers.

It doesn't take a leap of faith to make a connection between the escalating rate of mental illness and our progressively declining diet.

Occasionally, the stimulus-response-reward mechanism we fall heir to goes awry.[8] When someone remarks that we are getting fat, we change course and see eating as a punishment rather than a reward. We think the solution is simply to avoid the foods that have accumulated fat on our bodies and go on a diet. Unless we reeducate our eating habit, however, our withdrawal symptoms become so overwhelming that we are lured back to our bad habits like a remote-controlled robot.

In some people, especially young women, this pleasure-punishment response can get out of hand and produce a catch-22 cycle of starvation diets, food binges, and damaging purges. The Cornell University psychologists who first identified this syndrome also gave it a name: bulimarexia, which is more commonly known as bulimia. People who suffer from bulimia are obsessed with body image and want to get slimmer to conform with contemporary ideals. To this end, they go on punishing crash diets (see Chapter 2) that deprive them of the sugary and buttery foods that created their weight problem. Their cravings increase with the intensity of the diet until they no longer can do without their addictions. The physical and psychological stresses of withdrawal trigger binges of their favorite foods.[9]

Bulimics seem to be so addicted to sweets that they have no natural limits on the amounts they consume. A typical food binge might include a dozen doughnuts, a pint or quart of ice cream, a pound of candy, or an entire chocolate cake. Bulimics then force themselves to vomit and/or take a powerful laxative, then return to starving. Out of guilt, they begin an even more stringent diet.

Binging is not exclusive to bulimics, however. With so much refined sugar added to such ordinary diet staples as green beans, tomato sauce, bread, and salt (yes, sugar is added to some brands of salt, allegedly to keep it free-flowing), we are binging daily. Sugar is such an ingrained American habit that it may be impossible to ever remove it from our food supply. Your only alternative then is to do what you can to remove it from *your* food supply.

6

Sugar Stress

"The body does not lie. If you take sugar, you feel the consequences."

—*William Dufty*

SUGAR MANUFACTURERS urge us to eat sugar for a quick pick-me-up, thereby luring the unwary into a nutritional one-way street whose ultimate exit may be a stop called "sweet suicide." True, sugar does produce a rush of quick energy by raising your blood sugar level, but it falls just as abruptly a short time later. Sugar is absorbed into the bloodstream within minutes of being ingested, but within half an hour or so the energy is used up and you are probably left with the familiar symptoms of your descent from a sugar "high": irritability, dizziness, a headache, an inability to concentrate, or sleepiness and fatigue.[1]

What this plunge in your blood sugar level has done is to send shock waves through every cell in the body, especially the nervous system and the brain. To handle this sudden overdose of sugar, the body responds with its own overdose of insulin, a reaction doctors call insulin overshoot. Insulin is a hormone whose function is to remove excess sugar from the blood by sending it to body cells to be used as energy or stored as fat. This overreaction is a natural response that has its origins in our evolutionary past, when the only significant sugar we ate came from fruits and vegetables.

When we eat a piece of candy or a chocolate chip cookie, the body is, in effect, tricked into expecting to process carbohydrates, fats, protein, fiber, and other components of a whole food. In its natural past the body had never experienced a dose of sugar in its pure chemical state, so it releases a large shot of insulin to handle the meal the sugar indicates is present. With too much sugar being cleared from the bloodstream, the result is a drop to below-normal blood sugar levels, initiating a craving for more sweets, along with a host of physical and mental symptoms.[2]

About 10 percent of the population is said to suffer from a chronic and severe form of low blood sugar called hypoglycemia. This estimate is considered conservative by some nutritionists, however, and a great many more of us are likely to be suffering from milder forms of the condition.[3]

When blood sugar levels decline rapidly, the first organ to feel the effect is the brain. While other parts of the body can break down fats and protein to use as fuel, the brain relies on sugar processed by other organs to function properly. When deprived of its fuel, the brain begins to go haywire, and if the condition is not corrected the patient may faint and even go into a coma. The standard treatment in emergency rooms, in fact, is an intravenous injection of glucose solution.

In trying to correct its problem of low blood sugar, the body calls into play the adrenal glands, which stimulate the liver and muscles into releasing some of their stored sugar to bring up the blood sugar level. It's this release of adrenaline that causes many of the symptoms of a hypoglycemia attack. Adrenaline can cause heart palpitations and, by closing small blood vessels in the skin, produce the familiar cold sweat that anticipates the onset of hypoglycemia.

To diagnose abnormally low blood sugar, doctors rely on a procedure called the oral glucose tolerance test. The patient prepares himself by fasting the night before. Then in the morning he drinks a glucose solution that causes an immediate increase in blood sugar levels. The patient's blood sugar level is measured every five hours while insulin is being secreted. Hypoglycemia is indicated if, during this time, the patient's blood sugar level drops below normal while he simultaneously experiences the symptoms of hypoglycemia. If the test is inconclusive, the doctor may decide to monitor the patient's blood sugar level during the course of a normal day.

The same test is used to diagnose diabetes, which is the opposite of hypoglycemia. Diabetics suffer from hyperglycemia, which means there is too much sugar circulating in the blood and not enough insulin to handle it. Occasionally, a diabetic will take too high a dosage of medication, producing the nervous sweat and tingling tongue that signals hypoglycemia. Unless the diabetic has on hand a lump of sugar or a heavily sweetened food when the symptoms begin, the attack may result in loss of consciousness and even death.

Most Americans travel through life on a sugar roller coaster, attributing generalized symptoms to overwork or the inevitable process of aging. When we complain of episodic jitters and irritability to our doctors, they usually neglect the underlying causes and prescribe tranquilizers, beginning, for some, another pattern of addiction. When we complain of lassitude or boredom, doctors often advise eating something sweet to bring up our energy level— thus refueling the roller coaster's engines.

When we go to work on clogged highways or crowded public transportation systems, when we deal with cantankerous colleagues and customers, when we agonize over earning more money than we did the year before, we are making hefty withdrawals from our endocrine banks. Our bodies are continually begging for adrenaline to cope with the stresses of contemporary life. Throughout the day we crave pick-me-ups from coffee, tea, candy bars, sweet rolls, soft drinks, alcoholic beverages, and cigarettes. More coffee, another doughnut, maybe a cigarette, and the victim feels calm enough to endure until it's time for a high-carbohydrate lunch and soft drink. By three o'clock, the victim is tense and irritable, anticipating the afternoon coffee wagon and its array of tempting goodies. Exhausted by quitting time, he or she can't get home fast enough for another soft drink or a cocktail.

As with refined sugar, stress and stimulants also trigger an adrenal shock response. In addition, stress depletes the body of vitamin C and the B vitamins, both of which are required by the adrenal glands to function properly. The B complex group is essential to metabolizing the sugar you've inflicted on yourself. But since the B vitamins were stripped from the sugar during the refining process, there is none to help do the job. To make matters worse, caffeine in the coffee you've drunk is also calling on the adrenals to mobilize the body's energy reserves.[4]

Eventually, the adrenals become so overworked by these daily emergencies that they lose some of their ability to cope. Insulin secretion becomes imbalanced and you have on your hands a systemic problem involving the pancreas, adrenal glands, and liver. In some cases of excessive insulin secretion (hyperinsulinism), the body greatly reduces its sensitivity to the hormone. This may create a prediabetic condition in which the excess sugar stays in the blood long enough to do damage before glucose metabolism begins. These prediabetics are prone to cataracts, thickening of kidney membranes, nerve damage, and a decline in the capacity of the blood to carry oxygen throughout the body.

In 1973 the AMA labeled hypoglycemia a "nondisease," despite the fact that it has been shown to be a common denominator in many misdiagnosed patients. What prompted the AMA to come to this conclusion was a fad for self-diagnosis that followed the publication of several nutrition books in the 1960s and 1970s that attributed any number of ills to hypoglycemia. Doctors reported that many patients complaining of low blood sugar actually were suffering from emotional problems. Most of these patients were not considered hypoglycemics because they failed to show clinical symptoms when given the oral glucose tolerance test.

Recent research, however, supports the view that a milder degree of low blood sugar levels is widespread. Hypoglycemia never was a disease, of course: it is a symptom of a hormone imbalance which indicates that many glands and organs are not functioning properly. A study published in 1981 in *Orthomolecular Psychology* connects this imbalance to a surprising number of emotional and physical disorders, including schizophrenia, anxiety, chronic fatigue, the inability to concentrate, and a number of allergies. According to the study, the current upsurge in drug addiction, antisocial behavior, and criminality may be due, in some measure, to the junk diet that the present generation of youths was nurtured on.[5]

Because they eat the wrong foods and saturate themselves with sugar, many young people are apparently growing up brain-starved. Every time teenagers drink a can of soda, they are driving up their blood sugar levels, bringing insulin into play to clear out the glucose—and thereby depriving the brain of adequate nutrition. To understand how this works, you have to know that the brain has two basic parts, the cortex and the thalamus. Our primitive emotions of aggression, anger, and survival originate in the thalamus, which is all we have going for us when we are born. The process of emotional maturation is the work of the cortex, the outer layer of the brain, which gradually changes us from selfish little animals into civilized human beings.

We may want to strike out at those who are unfair to us, but the thinking cortex says no: the crime of assault may result in the loss of a job, a jail sentence, and the disapproval of others. Therefore, for our—and society's—greater good, we grin and bear it. Similarly, we may be tempted by the false nirvana of drugs or to steal what we can't afford, but our intellectual selves think better of it. It may well be, in the opinion of some, that glucose malnourishments upset the delicate compromise between the cortex and thalamus. In particularly frustrated individuals the effect may be even stronger. As the late nutritionist Carlton Fredericks pointed out, low blood sugar is "an excellent example not only of the influence of mind on body, but of the reverse equation often neglected: the influence of body on mind."[6]

Controlling low blood sugar is easier said than done, however, given the all-pervasive use of sugar in our food supplies. If you have been eating lots of sugar and white flour for years, you may have to forswear all sweet things for the rest of your life. Experiments with rats fed refined carbohydrates until they developed hypoglycemia showed that the symptoms ended once the offending foods were removed. But as soon as they returned to their old diet, the symptoms came back in force. Once the pancreas has been sensitized to sugar, it can never again tolerate large doses of it.[7]

If you are not that far gone, you can probably abort your journey to an assortment of debilitating ailments. Nutritionists place the reduction of stress first on the list, not only to reduce drain on the adrenals but to ease the craving for sweets which stress engenders. Avoiding *all* refined carbohydrates comes next. In addition to sugar and honey, that includes *all* products to which they have been added, even in minute amounts (to counter a cumulative effect); all products made with devitalized white flour, including noodles, white bread, biscuits, rolls, and crackers; and all beverages containing caffeine. Until your system readjusts, you also should cut down on fruit and fruit juice, and dried fruits. These contain a great percentage of natural sugars, and you should take them only in the presence of other foods, as with a meal.

In brief, a low blood sugar diet should be relatively high in protein, moderate in fats and complex carbohydrates, and low in natural sugars. In about a week or two, you should be able to resume eating fruit and fruit products, and to add more complex carbohydrates to your diet. You will be surprised at how alert and vital you feel once you have conquered the sugar monster. If you suspect you have the clinical form of hypoglycemia, you should, of course, take the glucose tolerance test.

7

Grazing in the Wrong Pastures

"Food is an important part of a balanced diet."
—*Fran Lebowitz*

TWENTY YEARS AGO it seemed that we were on the verge of a nutritional new age, one in which consumers would bring agri-businesses and food conglomerates to heel by demanding whole foods unadulterated by refined sugar, salt, chemical additives, fertilizers, and pesticides. Today, although we still pay lip service to this goal, it remains an elusive hope for the future.

Sugar is no longer high on our list of concerns, however, if it is included at all. The millions of dollars spent by the Sugar Association have finally paid off, and most people have been convinced that if sugar isn't exactly good for us, it isn't bad for us either. For those with a lingering doubt, food processors brazenly assure us we have all cut down by minimally reducing sugar in a few products that were overloaded with sugar to begin with.

Ironically, those of us with the worst eating habits are the so-called baby boomers, who have probably been exposed to more information about nutrition than any other generation in history. But this is also the same generation reared by working mothers and fathers, whose babysitter was often a can of soda, a bag of cookies, and a television set. When mom and dad were too tired to prepare a proper meal, there was always a fast-food outlet nearby to provide a cheap and convenient substitute.

During nearly two decades following World War II, some 73 million babies were born in the United States, the largest population bubble ever. Dubbed the "baby boom generation," they have within their brief history been labeled the "TV generation," the "now generation," the "me generation," and "the Pepsi generation." But whatever they are called, baby boomers have to a large degree reshaped America's eating patterns. Raised during a period of unprecedented economic growth, they have enjoyed a luxury of choice unknown to previous generations—in careers, marital arrangements, recreation, and, especially, in food and drink.

When boomers began to come of age in the late 1960s, they promised to become the most physically fit and nutritionally aware generation of Americans we have ever known. "Revolution," a buzzword of the 1960s and early 1970s, was also meant to include a revolution in the health of our bodies and the quality of the foods we put into them. Sugar became a no-no and for a brief period—from 1972 to 1975—our per capita consumption actually decreased when the price shot up.[1] Strenuous physical exercise was on everyone's mind, and soon streets and parks everywhere were filled with joggers and runners.

Meanwhile, after its short-lived setback, sugar and its caloric siblings were once again insinuating themselves into the American diet. While we had all cut back on table sugar, reducing our average per capita intake by nearly thirty pounds per year, we had in fact begun to eat more sugar than ever before. From 1975 to 1987 we increased our annual consumption from 118 pounds per person annually to more than 130 pounds. Many of us, boomers in particular, had fallen off the wagon and succumbed to that fondly remembered candy-coated teat of our childhoods.[2] Moreover, as the baby boom generation approached middle age, it was losing interest in physical fitness.

"Exercise is out," *The Wall Street Journal* reported in a front-page article in January 1989. In a survey of the fitness industry, the *Journal* found that health clubs were losing members by the score, and that the number of people who ran, swam, played tennis, or did calisthenics had declined by 5 percent to 20 percent between 1984 and 1987. The paper concluded that "for many yuppies—the prime movers in the fitness boom—exercise is becoming boring."[3]

The good news was that there are still a significant number of Americans who exercise, although not with the same evangelical fervor as before. Cycling has shown an increase, according to the National Sporting Goods Association, as has exercise walking, which gained seventeen million new fans in the period between 1984 and 1987. The trend is definitely away from regular workouts, however, which are giving way to the occasional half hour of exercise, or, for a growing number of boomers, no exercise at all.

At the same time, boomers are eating more candy, ice cream, cookies, salty snack foods, and beef, and, consequently, putting on weight. In the past, these trends would have signaled an increase in people on diets, but the number of Americans attempting to reduce their weight actually has declined. The NPD Group, a Chicago-based market research company which analyzes American eating habits, surveyed 2,000 households from 1984 to 1986 and found that the number of dieters had fallen from 27 percent to 19 percent. MRCA Information Services, another marketing research firm, coincidentally discovered in its own study that from 1980 to 1985 dieters had just about doubled their intake of chocolate candy, sweetened breakfast rolls, and other high-calorie goodies.[4]

These studies demonstrate just how ineffective most diets are and how difficult they are to stay with. But more to the point, they show how important it is to first kick the sugar habit before attempting to slim down. Without this first step, a dieter will inevitably succumb to the insatiable cravings engendered by a lifetime of sugar addiction.

Nestled among baby boomers, at the visible end of the scale, are the yuppies, young urban professionals, who toil in select white-collar jobs and whose income is well above the national average. Judging from their education level (many have advanced college degrees) and the sophisticated work they perform, not to mention their disposable income, one would think that yuppies would be extraordinarily discriminating in the food and beverages they buy. What they choose, however, is not much different from what less-distinguished boomers prefer: it is merely more expensive.

With cash to spend—and an eagerness to spend it—yuppies have become a prime target of the food and beverage industries, which perceive them as setting trends for fellow boomers. Yuppies spend lots of credit-card money eating out, prompting many restauranteurs to accommodate them with menus reminiscent of foods they enjoyed as children. It is to well-heeled boomers that we owe the new fad of grazing, which is to select small portions of items on the menu because we like them, which is rather like choosing one's dinner as a series of snacks. And what tastes good is usually synonymous with what tastes sweet, rich, and salty.

Dessert (and there is always room for more sugar) may be a slice of chocolate–peanut butter pie, which resembles Reese's Peanut Butter Cups; "Death by Chocolate" cake, a sugar-saturated, butter-soaked gourmet version of chocolate pudding; or that old standby S'mores, a gooey concoction of melted chocolate, graham crackers, and marshmallows, best enjoyed as a childhood memory.

A leading exponent of grazing was the late artist Andy Warhol, whose personal style provided an aesthetic for thousands of yuppies. "I'll buy a huge piece of meat, cook it up for dinner," Warhol once told a magazine interviewer, "then right before it's done, I'll break down and have what I wanted for dinner in the first place—bread and jam . . . all I ever really want is sugar."[5] In 1987 Warhol's poisonous diet and sedentary life-style finally caught up with him, and he entered New York Hospital to have his gall bladder removed. Complications followed the routine surgery, however, and Warhol died at the age of sixty-one in his hospital bed.

Whatever the immediate cause of Warhol's death, it seems likely the pasty-faced, white-haired artist had seriously impaired his immune system and his capacity for recovery. Gallbladder disease and gallstones are another disease of civilization caused primarily by eating too many refined carbohydrates, saturated fats, and dairy products such as ice cream, and not enough fiber and foods rich in vitamin E, lecithin, vitamin C, and the vitamin B complex. The function of the gallbladder, a small saclike organ behind the liver, is to collect the bile produced by the liver and concentrate it for later use in digesting fats. Sugar, refined carbohydrates, and saturated fats tax the gallbladder's efforts to help digest and absorb fats (including the fat-soluble vitamins E and A), and decrease the bile flow. As a result, natural bile acids are no longer available to the body in amounts necessary to lower cholesterol. The majority of gallstones are in fact composed largely of cholesterol crystals. Extremely painful, a gallbladder attack usually comes on without warning as a knife-like pain in the upper right abdomen, often spreading to the back and right shoulder. Millions of Americans are said to be harboring silent gallstones that will not show symptoms for many years.

Interestingly, after Warhol's premature death, collectors eager to own a piece of the artist paid tens of thousands of dollars for his collection of cookie jars. While these vintage jars may indicate

Warhol's unerring eye for collectibles, they can also be seen as a reminder of the folly of living life as a sugar junkie.

One of the greatest merchandising successes of the decade has been "designer" ice creams laced with crumbled candy or cookies. The market leaders are vanilla flavors mixed with Oreo cookie pieces or Heath Bar chips.[6] The makers of Oreo cookies and Heath Bars have found a new demand for their products while also finding a convenient means of disposal for cookies and candy bars broken on the assembly line. Such a combination packs a powerful caloric wallop and, as the old joke goes, you may as well "just glue it to your hips" rather than bothering to eat it. Even without the candy or cookies, designer ice creams, which are denser and contain more butterfat than the usual supermarket variety, have about 300 calories per one-cup serving. Add to that the empty calories of half of a Heath Bar and you bring the total up to about 375.

The latest upscale sweet to hit supermarket shelves is white chocolate.[7] For those willing to take the risk, there are Nestlé's Alpine White bar, the company's biggest seller since its Crunch bar, white chocolate chip cookies, Duncan Hines's Vienna White brownie mix, white chocolate filled pasta, and even white chocolate flavored toothpaste. Campbell Soup's Godiva subsidiary reports that sales are booming for its Ivory White chocolate, which at $28 a pound may buy status but not good health. The only advantage to white chocolate—and it is a negative plus—is its lack of theobromine and caffeine, stimulants that cause reactions in those allergic to ordinary chocolate.

Sad to say, an entire generation of well-educated Americans is backsliding into a nutritional abyss that can only lead to health problems in later life. While boomers profess to want nutritious food, statistics show they are not eating as well as their elders. Candy consumption has gone up by more than three pounds per person in this decade,[8] and, according to the Department of Commerce, the American obsession with ice cream is at an all-time record level. Snacking at home is on the increase as are take-out fast foods.

What younger Americans apparently want today are familiar, comforting foods that don't need to be cooked and are delivered to them in the most convenient way possible. When the NPD Group began its survey, a majority of respondents put nutrition at the top of their list; by 1986 most householders had changed their minds and put convenience first. Only 22 percent still believed that nutrition was the most important consideration.

With more and more Americans eating on the run, you can be sure that food companies are not lagging behind. "Convenience is not enough anymore," said a spokesman—prophetically in 1987—for Product Initiatives, one of the processed food industry's most prestigious consultants. "It is very important for food to be in smaller portions, to be a one-person or one-occasion size offering. The leading edge is that it is hand-held food."[9]

Since then, food manufacturers and fast food restaurants have taken their sweet snacks and desserts out of dishes, bowls, and glasses and frozen them onto sticks or sealed them into plastic containers and Mylar bags. The breakthrough had come several years before, when General Foods, the industry leader, transformed its Jell-O pudding into Jell-O Pudding Pops, a major success that prompted the giant food conglomerate to premix Kool-Aid powder and put it into single-serving containers. Nabisco was quick to follow by repackaging Oreo cookies and its Fig Newtons in small sizes. Lipton then came along with individual pie servings sold under its Country Inn label. Tally these products up with all the Popsicles, ice cream bars, and frozen yogurt bars that have long been available in supermarket freezers and you have a numbing variety of sugar-on-a-stick items to choose from.

Since nutritionists had been aware that America's eating habits had long gone from promising to poor, they were not very surprised when *The New York Times* revealed in 1988 the results of a nutrition poll of 1,870 people. "Instead of teaching good nutrition in schools," commented Bonnie Liebman, director of nutrition at the Center for Science in the Public Interest, a consumer advocacy group based in Washington, D.C., "we subject our kids to television commercials that push fast foods, soft drinks, candy bars, and sugary cereals. And then we wonder why kids don't ask for fruits and vegetables."[10]

What the *Times* determined in its poll was that few people of any age have heeded the call to better nutrition. Candy, baked goods, ice cream, and frozen desserts topped the list of preferred in-between foods, followed by potato chips and corn chips, popcorn and peanuts, with fresh fruit, juice, and vegetables trailing in a distant third place. The group who indulged themselves the most were eighteen- to forty-four-year-olds, an age group that would include baby boomers as well as some of their children. Older, and wiser perhaps, forty-five- to sixty-four-year-olds ate fewer (but still too many) sugars and starches, while those over sixty-four, the boomers' grandparents, consumed the least and were the most likely to choose a piece of fruit, juice, and milk, cheese, or yogurt.

8

The Fast-Food Lane

"Got to be mighty careful when you're eatin' out."
—*Colonel Sanders*

ALL ROADS eventually lead to fast foods today. Millions of Americans plunk down billions of dollars every year at 200,000 fast food restaurants across the nation, where we line up in fake villas, plaster rancheros, and plastic roadside palaces waiting to buy hamburgers, French fries, milkshakes, tacos, pizzas, croissant sandwiches, barbecued ribs, cheap steaks—you name it. Fifteen years ago there were fewer than 30,000 of these cheapjack establishments, and fewer than half of all Americans who eat out took meals there. By 1987 that figure had risen to over 75 percent of all Americans.[1]

America's journey to the fast food wonderland has been a comparatively rapid one made possible by the proliferation of the automobile and the development of thousands of miles of interlocking freeways. It all began around the turn of the century with the invention of the hamburger, either at New Haven's Louis Lunch diner in 1900 or at the 1904 St. Louis World's Fair.[2] (Gastronomic historians have yet to determine which claim is true.) But it was at the St. Louis Fair that two other easily prepared, portable food items were introduced: the ice cream cone and iced tea.

By the 1930s thousands of motorized Americans were slowly

but surely altering the country's eating habits. Speed and convenience seemed ideally suited to a population increasingly on the move. Hamburger stands proliferated, followed by fancier drive-ins that offered attractive carhops who delivered your beefburger, wimpeyburger, steerburger, White Castle burger, or what have you to your dining room cum automobile.

But it took the marketing genius of an ex-Sears salesman named Ray Kroc to transform the hamburger into a product that is endlessly replicable. Kroc simply transferred his expertise in marketing cheap clothing, dishes, musical instruments, and furniture to marketing cheap food and drink to the same mass market. Profit margins were increased by doing away with carhops and having customers serve themselves. Cost control was imperative: hamburgers were measured to the last ounce, customers always got the same amount of French fries, and milkshakes were automatically dispensed, leaving virtually no chance for error. These technical innovations made it possible for Kroc's McDonald's chain to hire cheap inexperienced help such as high school students, since very little judgment was required to serve the customer.[3]

Although Kroc is no longer with us, his name lives on in the annals of American business, and of course in the golden arches that dot our visually polluted highways. We can also thank Kroc for all the other fast food chains that have followed in McDonald's wake.

Americans believe they frequent these glittering nutritional traps because they are cheap and convenient. But there is a more pervasive reason: Fast food chains keep customers coming back for more because their fare is loaded with addictive sugar, fat, and salt. And, as had happened with Coca-Cola, the fast food habit is rapidly spreading throughout the industrialized world.

True, eating at Burger King or Pizza Hut is incredibly convenient. The limited menu requires a minimum of decision-making, and there is no need to shop for groceries, cook them, and wash the dishes. The meals are filling, and less than $5 will buy a double-cheeseburger, or a large slice of sausage pizza, and French fries, a milkshake, or a Coke.

You get a lot for your money, but you also get large helpings of overnutrition and malnutrition. The USDA's dietary survey indicates that the number of Americans who ate an adequately nutritious diet actually declined between 1955 and 1985—the same period in which fast food franchisers changed our eating habits.

The problem built into most fast food meals is that they are still not nutritionally balanced. While there is more than enough protein per meal, there are too many sugar and fat calories and salt, and not enough vitamins, minerals, and fiber. You've probably gotten your entire carbohydrate (sugar and starch) allowance, and if you're driving there's no opportunity to work it off.

The total calorie count of a typical fast food meal consisting of a cheeseburger with the works, French fries, and a milkshake totals approximately 1,300, or half the daily ration required for an adult male. If you ate such a meal every day—while consuming two other meals—you would gain weight. Women would put on even more pounds since their caloric requirements are lower.

All fast foods are presalted, and *Consumer Reports* magazine found that the average sodium content of eight meals tested was well over a teaspoonful—and that does not include table salt many people sprinkle on their food.[4] That's nearly a full day's supply for a person on the mildest of salt-restricted diets. More than half the calories in a fast food meal come from fat, which takes care of your allowance for the day. And then there are those sixteen to twenty teaspoons of sugar which are in the hamburger bun, the cheese, the special sauce, ketchup, and Coke, or milkshake.

In recent years it has become the fashion among some nutritionists (fast-food merchandisers employ powerful public relations

agencies) to minimize the risks and exaggerate the benefits of a fast
food meal. You can get a nutritious meal at your local foodstand,
they claim, if you refrain from the special sauce, don't order
French fries, and drink milk or water instead of a sugared soft drink
or a prefabricated milkshake. Another important caveat is not to
rely on fast foods as your major meal. No one can quarrel with these
arguments, but they entirely miss the point. Fast food chains are
in business to sell the entire package, and they are constantly
wooing the consumer with discount tie-ins (''French fries or Coke
free with a double whamburger''), coupons, contests (''peel open
a ticket and win a fortune!''), slapstick movies, and lovable
clowns.

Long before you first entered a McDonald's or Wendy's or
Burger King, the creators of these institutions were well aware of
your food addictions. They knew that (1) you prefer the sweet,
bland, and mildly sour, and (2) you would not wait for more than
six minutes to taste what you hungered for. Ray Kroc found this
out when he studied government figures on what a typical American eats every year. Back then it was only 100 pounds of sugar,
55 pounds of fats and oils, 400 cans of soft drinks, 30 gallons of
ice cream, 8 pounds of potato chips, 63 dozen doughnuts, 60
pounds of cookies and cakes, 40 pounds of chopped meat, and
more than 200 pounds of candy, popcorn, pies, and assorted snacks
laden with fat and sugar.[5]

Ten years ago the American Psychiatric Association published
a report that clearly defined the appeal of fast foods:

> The right feeling of food in the mouth is avidly pursued by
> fast food purveyors. It cues past association from our child-
> hood when our food habits were formed. There is already a
> need for the crispy and crunchy, for the over-sweet and the
> unsophisticated ''usual.''

Fast food professionals know that in America fondness for the undistinguished in food is a national trait linked with what appears to be safe and wholesome.

This provides the answer why fast food franchises are so successful. Their limited menus of carbohydrate bulk, with fat, are monotonously unpretentious. The hamburger, chicken, etc. are prepared in the same familiar assembly-line style of the food from the freezer, the can, or the plastic pouch. It reminds them of "home"—up-to-date style. Millions rush to the fast food emporiums not so much because they are fast, but because these millions feel sure about what they are going to get.[6]

"Life is a chemical process," said Antoine-Laurent Lavoisier, the father of modern chemistry, two hundred years ago. And, he might have added were he alive today, if you want to keep your chemistry in balance, stay away from fast food restaurants. It was Lavoisier's experiments that led to the science of nutrition a century later. We now know for certain that for food to sustain human life and health, two needs have to be met: you need enough food to grow and provide your energy requirements; you must have specific nutrients within that food supply. In other words, we can become ill from not eating enough food and from eating food with not enough of the nutrients our bodies need.

The six essential nutrients commonly in short supply in fast food meals are the B vitamins folacin, biotin, pantothenic acid, all of vitamin A, and the minerals iron and copper. These perform a variety of life-sustaining tasks.[7] For B vitamins to be completely absorbed, all the other B vitamins must be present. Each member of the vitamin B complex has a distinct function in maintaining the digestive and nervous systems, and in reducing the accumulation of cholesterol. Others help convert food into energy, and keep the heart and muscles in good shape.

A U.S. Department of Agriculture survey released in 1985 indicated that the calcium, zinc, and iron intakes of teenage girls—a great many of whom are members of the fast food generation—were less than two-thirds of the Recommended Daily Allowance. Young adult women fared better on calcium intake, but they were getting even less iron and zinc than their younger counterparts. The study declared that the intake of the trace mineral copper fell below ''estimated safe and adequate'' levels.

The nutritional scheme of trace minerals is not yet entirely understood, but it is known that they often act in tandem with major minerals. Copper, for example, assists iron in carrying oxygen to the cells of the body. And zinc and manganese are needed if calcium is to build strong bones and prevent osteoporosis.[8] Low levels of trace minerals therefore may prevent the body from working at optimum capacity, which can translate into sluggishness and impaired mental performance.

Directly affected by a high consumption of sugar is chromium, which helps the hormone insulin regulate blood sugar levels. ''Drinking a sugar soda after eating a starchy meal and then ice cream smothered with chocolate fudge can drain your body of chromium,'' stated the Agricultural Research Service of the USDA in a report issued in the summer of 1989. To process a heavily sugared diet, the body requires more chromium than it would normally to keep blood sugar in check. Since sugar and starch lose natural chromium in the refining process, the body must pump out more and more insulin to process these foods, thereby taxing the body's fail-safe mechanism to keep blood glucose levels in balance. (See Chapter 6.) The more chromium the body uses, the more it loses—and it is not likely to be replaced by the semisynthetic diet of a sugar addict.

Vitamin A, which is stored in body fat, is not found in nature as is. To get enough of it, you have to eat a lot of pigmented vegetables like carrots and broccoli, or fish, liver, and milk so that the body will have enough beta-carotene to manufacture it. Burger fanciers who don't eat enough of these foods may be in store for bouts of night blindness, respiratory infections, and the fatigue that accompanies anemia. Deficiencies in iron and copper also contribute to these conditions, but if you get your quota of beta-carotene you'll ingest more than enough of these minerals.

Pizza remains the safest buy in a fast-food restaurant. Pizza is high in protein, comparatively low in fat, and offers the fewest calories you can get in a fast-food chain. A vegetarian topping of tomato sauce, green pepper, onions, and mushrooms boosts vitamin, mineral, and fiber content, but there may be as much as a teaspoon of sugar in the tomato sauce. Pizza is also highest in salt content, making it a risky investment for millions of Americans developing high blood pressure from their diets and life-styles—particularly for those over age fifty. Anyone already diagnosed with hypertension should stay away from *all* fast foods because they contain so much sodium that the chance of a premature heart attack or stroke is enhanced.

Customers at Wendy's, McDonald's, Pizza Hut, and their siblings might make wiser choices if all the ingredients in their foods were listed on the menu board, as they are by law in fast food restaurants in West Germany. Honest labeling hasn't dampened profits in that country, where components in food items, whether packaged in supermarkets or served in restaurants, must be clearly identified. In the United States, many chains publish booklets revealing how much sugar, fat, and salt is in their foods, but try and find one. They're allegedly available in the restaurants, but recent requests in several outlets were met with blank stares by the staff who were apparently unaware these exist.

Instead of helping us make educated choices, the fast-food industry prefers to spend its advertising and public relations budget enticing us into the symbolic golden arch. In 1988, the Marriott Corporation, owner of the Roy Rogers fast food chain, launched an ad campaign that appeared to praise junk food at the expense of a nutritious meal. In the widely seen television commercial, actors dressed as cafeteria servers offered students trays of unappealing gray glop in a school lunchroom. The commercial then flashed to delectable visions of lunches available at Roy Rogers franchises. Marriott claimed the commercial was meant to be funny and nothing more, but not everyone got the joke. Amid complaints from consumer groups and parents, it withdrew the ad.[9]

Even though we know better, commercials like these tend to shout down low-profile nutritionists who tell us it just ain't so. As fast food outlets continue to expand, it seems likely that fewer and fewer of us will attempt to reconcile our wants with our needs.

9

The Osteoporosis Explosion

"All tastes are acquired tastes. We are born with a taste for nothing except human milk."

—*Euell Gibbons*

THE WORD *osteoporosis* conjures up images of an elderly man or woman, back stooped in a deformed curve, balance unsteady. For most Americans, osteoporosis is a malady of then, not of now, to be faced when the time comes. Rarely, if at all, do we think of it in terms of a younger generation—our children—let alone consider the possibility they will inherit an epidemic of this painful, debilitating condition.

Osteoporosis means "porous bone," and it refers to a loss of tissue that causes the bones to shrink and become increasingly brittle. Symptoms of the disorder include pains in the hip and back, and reduced height. As the condition progresses, a simple fall or bump, or merely lifting a small package can snap a wrist, thigh, or hip bone like a dried twig, necessitating a long and expensive hospital stay in traction. Incredibly, some fifteen to twenty million Americans currently suffer from weakened bone structures, which medical experts claim are a primary cause of the 1.3 million fractures that occur every year in people over forty-five.[1]

Bone, of course, is not an unalterably rigid substance. Osteoblast and osteoclast cells are constantly dissolving and reforming every bone in our skeletons every day. Like every other tissue in the body, there is no single bone strut that remains permanent. To maintain this complex biochemical process, however, we require a constant, fresh supply of calcium.

This vital mineral, acting in conjunction with vitamin D and phosphorus, not only builds and maintains bones and teeth, it is essential to healthy blood, a regular heartbeat, and even a good night's sleep. In addition, calcium helps convert food to energy and plays a part in muscle growth and in the transmission of nerve impulses. Of the twenty or so known minerals we need to live, calcium is the most abundant in our bodies, with about 99 percent of it contained in our bones and teeth.

While the recommended minimum daily requirement (MDR) for the average adult has been set at 800 milligrams (equivalent to the calcium in about two glasses of milk), estimates are that over 30 percent of Americans get 450 milligrams or less. In other words, a large—and growing—minority of Americans is suffering from calcium deficiency.[2]

What is so alarming about this statistic is that it points a finger at millions of teenagers whose growing bones require an even greater amount of calcium than their parents: 1,000 milligrams daily. Why aren't the children of the richest, most sophisticated food producer in the world getting all the milk they need? It's a question you might well ask. And the answer would be, in a word: sugar!

Traditionally, America's teenagers have been avid milk-drinkers, but within a generation they have begun to desert this wholesome food in favor of syrupy, nonnutritious carbonated soft drinks. According to industry figures, from 1970 to 1987 soft drink sales more than doubled, from 49.5 billion 12-ounce cans to nearly 120 billion. This translates into an increase from approximately 243 cans per year per American in 1970 to an astonishing 450 cans each today. Since these figures are averages based on an overall total, we can safely assume that because some people drink no carbonated sodas, others are downing many more than their statistical allotment of 1.2 cans per day.[3]

How endemic the addiction of teenagers to soft drinks has become was made apparent by a survey, published in 1986, of 4,455 representative adolescents. Conducted by Patricia M. Guenther, a nutrition analyst for the Agriculture Department, the study showed that teens who drank the most soft drinks also drank the least milk. Guenther's study further indicated that soft drinks had become for many the beverage of choice to accompany lunch and dinner—and even breakfast.

While most people still find the idea of Coke and oatmeal for breakfast ludicrous, a great many others do not. According to the National Soft Drink Association, Americans drink four times more canned soda than fruit juice, and 12 percent of these soft drinks are consumed for breakfast. The prospect of yet another empty food crowding out a nutritious one elicited a unanimous groan from nutritionists around the country, but at Coca-Cola headquarters in Atlanta, only sounds of rejoicing could be heard. "We're in the middle of a watershed movement," boasted a Coke spokesman to a *New York Times* reporter.[4] "The move toward soft drinks in the morning is clearly a social phenomenon." The Coke executive was interviewed shortly after the company announced plans to turn this unhealthy trend into a national habit with an advertising campaign whose slogan is "Coke in the Morning." As it had done successfully in the past in fast food outlets, the company hooks the consumer with a marketing technique known as "cross-merchandising." Cans of Coke, for example, are displayed prominently at a counter filled with commercial pastries over which a banner announces that the cola will be sold at discount to anyone who buys one of the sugary baked goods.

Marketing experts claim young Americans are switching to soft drinks for breakfast because the beverages are more compatible with current life-styles than are customary hot morning beverages. In an era when so many young people seem to be on the run, the thinking goes, it is more convenient to grab a can of soda from the refrigerator than to bother with pouring a glass of fruit juice and lighting the stove to prepare coffee, tea, or hot chocolate. This may well be true, but the soft drink habit has more to do with cleverly manipulative advertising campaigns than it has with conscious choice. In recent decades, soft drink companies have outspent all milk, fruit juice, and bottled water producers combined in pervasive advertising campaigns that ceaselessly encourage young people to swallow ever more of their products.

How effective these massive assaults are on our beverage habits is apparent from the per capita statistics we quoted above. Parents, themselves weaned on soft drinks a generation ago, see no harm in pacifying their toddlers with artificially colored, artificially flavored, and artificially carbonated sodas. As a result, 40 percent of the country's one- to two-year-olds now imbibe an average of nine ounces of soft drinks every day.[5] As they grow older, of course, they will, like their parents, drink more and more of these ghastly concoctions. Is it any wonder then that people between the ages of twenty-two and forty-four are the largest consumers of soft drinks, making up about 27 percent of the $38 billion a year market?[6]

One of Coca-Cola's advertisements, played on radio stations during peak commuting hours, urges drivers to stop for "a cool refreshing drink to make me come alive." But rather than quench thirst, soft drinks actually trigger a demand for sugar that leaves one thirstier for more of the same. What the consumer is actually buying is a convenient package that can be carried anywhere, with no preparation or cleaning up involved, to satisfy an addiction to intensely flavored sweetness. The best antidote to thirst remains plain old water.

While sodas have no real nutritive value, they do contain a number of undesirable ingredients which may be especially hazardous to growing young bodies. In addition to that seven to ten teaspoons of sugar in an average 12-ounce can, you are getting synthetic colorings, flavorings, and preservatives. While there are some soft drinks that are caffeine-free, most cola-based drinks contain significant amounts of this stimulant. One can of Dr. Pepper, for example, provides a child with as much as half the caffeine you get in your cup of coffee. Another undesirable ingredient is phosphoric acid, a cheaply produced acidulant used to bring out the cola flavor and add an agreeable tartness. The corrosive qualities of phosphoric acid are well known (drop a penny in a glass of cola and see what happens), and in large quantities it not only interferes with the absorption of calcium, it can corrode the teeth. At about thirty to eighty milligrams a can, sodium is not high, but when the cans start accumulating, so does the salt.

A new line of soft drinks labeled ''natural'' have recently been introduced to woo the nutrition-minded consumer. These may taste better because their flavors are from plant sources, but the colas and root beers contain as much caffeine as Coca-Cola and Tab. The sweetener used is fructose, which saves a few calories but is not significantly different from regular sugar.

And canned fruit drinks and ades aren't any better. These are really uncarbonated soft drinks, and mainly water, sugar, and additives to give the illusion of the real thing. If the manufacturer is being generous, he may even include as much as 10 percent fruit juice. At about a dollar a can or bottle of such a fruit drink, you will have to pay as much as $10 to get a full quart of juice.

The booby prize for sugared soft drinks has to go to Grape Tang.

You mix this dry purple powder with water, a process which allows a child to make the drink as sweet as he or she likes. The label says, in order of predominance, that it contains sugar, citric acid (for tartness), maltodextrin (provides body)—another sugar—calcium phosphates (regulates tartness and prevents caking), modified starches (provides body), vitamin C, natural flavors, xanthan gum (provides body), hydrogenated vegetable oils, artificial and natural colors, vitamin A palmitate, alpha tocopherol, and BHA (preservatives).

In 1980 the Food and Drug Administration issued a regulation requiring manufacturers of diluted juice drinks to state how much juice was in the can or jar. The food industry has many lobbyists in Washington, however, so the Reagan Administration was persuaded to put on hold indefinitely the deadline for compliance. Some companies have gone ahead and listed percentages on labels, however, but others have not. If it's called "juice cocktail," "juice drink," "fruit punch," or "juice blend," you're getting a diluted, heavily sweetened product. Pure juice has to be labeled "juice," although this is sometimes not the case. In 1987, a popular apple juice was found to contain only 10 percent apple juice; the rest was water and sugar.

Milk, a fluid secreted by the mammary glands of mammals to feed their young, remains the best source of calcium for most people. It's also a nearly complete food for infants and a highly nutritious complement to adult diets. Milk is a solution composed of butterfat, proteins, lactose (milk sugar), calcium, phosphorus, other minerals, and enzymes. The most important vitamins it contains are vitamins A and riboflavin, one of the B group, and vitamins C and E. Milk is usually fortified with added vitamin D to help the bones absorb calcium. Chocolate milk drinks may seem to be a happy compromise between a sweet tooth and a healthy body, but many of these prefabricated beverages contain too little milk and too much sugar and too many chemical additives to be healthful.

Some children and adults can't tolerate milk, however, not because they don't like it but because their small intestine lacks the enzyme necessary to break down lactose. When the lactose-intolerant drink milk they can become quite ill. Their stomachs become queasy and the result is often explosive diarrhea—and the consequent washing out of other nutrients before they are absorbed into the bloodstream. Americans of Mediterranean and African descent are most likely to have this disorder.

In the 1980s a number of supermarkets began carrying milk in which the lactose has been predigested. And, because their lactose has been converted by microorganism, cheese and yogurt will not upset a lactose-intolerant stomach.

There are about two and a half pounds of calcium in the body of a 160-pound man, about 99 percent of it stored in the bones and teeth. As a child grows, the need for calcium is at its highest point. During this phase, calcium is deposited in bone tissue faster than it is removed. We reach our skeletal peak—the time at which our bones are most dense and strong—at about age thirty-five in both men and women. After then, more calcium is lost than is replaced, and the bones gradually become less dense. Moreover, as men and women age, their bodies, for reasons not totally understood, are less efficient in absorbing calcium from food.

A certain amount of bone loss is inevitable for all of us, but osteoporosis—attenuated bone loss—doesn't have to be in our future. But for children growing up on sugary soft drinks just when they need calcium the most to build strong bones for a future, it may well be. One of those who has sounded the alarm is Jane E. Brody, nutrition columnist for *The New York Times*: "Given the status of calcium consumption among American teenagers, the osteoporosis epidemic could double or triple in size in the next generation."[7]

At present, the only treatment for this silent disease is to eat more calcium and to exercise more, both of which the patient probably didn't do much of earlier in life anyway. For postmenopausal women, more of whom are affected than middle-aged men, estrogen-replacement therapy can help decrease bone resorption. There are risks to this treatment, however. It increases the chance of uterine cancer, blood clots, and strokes.[8]

If you have grown up on an inadequate supply of protein, minerals, and vitamins, and continued to replace them with sugared and artificially sweetened nonfoods, then you may live to regret it. As nutritionist Dr. H. Curtis Wood, Jr., noted in his book *Overfed but Undernourished*: "Young people have an amazing ability to adjust and adapt to unbelievably deficient diets and yet feel fairly well. Because of this, they do not understand that while they may be able to get away with living on hamburgers, potato chips, and soda pop without apparent disastrous results for some years, it will eventually catch up with them in one way or another."

10

A Feast for Yeast

"What is food to one may be fierce poison to others."
—*Lucretius*

ONE OF OUR constant companions throughout life is a yeast organism called *Candida albicans*. Ordinarily, there aren't enough of these parasites inside our bodies to harm us, but in the last thirty years or so they have been making themselves feel more and more at home.

Also known as monilia, candida inhabits the skin, mouth, throat, intestines, and vagina. Most of the time it's kept under control by the body's defense barriers, but when the immune system is compromised the fungus can multiply and cause illness, which is why it is called an opportunistic infection.

When the disease strikes the mouth it produces ugly white patches on the tongue, often accompanied by fever. The condition, known as thrush, is all too familiar to doctors treating AIDS patients. Candida's favored home is the reproductive organs, however, especially those of the female. Harbored in the warm, moist environment of the vagina, candida, left unchecked, invades the vaginal tissues producing painful swelling, severe itching and/or a burning sensation, and an irritating discharge.[1]

Diabetics are particularly susceptible to yeast infections, as are cancer patients undergoing chemotherapy and those whose immune systems have been similarly compromised. Fortunately, for most women the causes of this nagging, often chronic condition are not life-threatening diseases but contemporary food and drug habits that can be altered with a little savvy and a lot of will power.

Some researchers refer to candida as the "twentieth-century disease" because they believe it is brought on by antibiotics, pollutants, and birth control pills, and fed by sugars and refined carbohydrates. The first to discover this missing link was Dr. C. Orian Truss, a Birmingham, Alabama, physician who is generally regarded as a pioneer in the study of the far-reaching effects of candida infections. According to Truss, when the fungus is out of balance, it causes symptoms that can be as varied as lethargy, fatigue, depression, mental confusion, headaches, hyperactivity, difficulty in breathing, and gastric and bowel problems.[2]

In his book *The Missing Diagnosis,* Dr. Truss details these symptoms and how they wax and wane in intensity, making it difficult for physicians to diagnose the condition. Consequently, states Truss, most doctors overlook the real cause. Instead, they diagnose the illness according to which organ—the heart, liver, pancreas, kidneys, whatever—is presently showing the most severe symptoms. Taking a culture is of little help since candida is a normal inhabitant of the body. The only accurate diagnosis is to study the patient's case history and to try out a treatment regime. If the treatment works, you've got, or had, candidiasis.

Truss's efforts in deciphering this diagnostic conundrum have spawned a large body of research on the subject, which is intriguingly detailed in *The Yeast Connection,* a cautionary overview by Dr. William G. Crook. In 1979, after frustrating years of being unable to cure an increasing number of patients with multiple complaints, Dr. Crook consulted with Dr. Truss, who advised him to treat these patients with a special diet, food supplements, and, if they needed it, a safe antifungal prescription medication called nystatin. "Almost without exception," Dr. Crook writes enthusiastically, "they improved. And some improved dramatically."

What the good doctors' clinical experience taught them is that candida is not mutating into a stronger strain; rather, it is we ourselves who are compromising our ability to fend it off. In a healthy individual, a trillion highly specialized cells, with hundreds of millions of years of evolutionary experience behind them, stand at the ready to repel any alien organism attempting to take over the body. With the voraciousness of Pac-Man, they gobble up any microbe that threatens to make us sick. When all systems are not go, normally dormant parasites in the body become active, and invaders have a field day.

When it comes to candida, the doctors say, even a minor compromise of the immune system can give rise to an attack of candidiasis. Our environment is saturated with chemical pollutants that weaken our ability to fight disease while at the same time triggering allergic reactions in many of us. Chemicals singled out include lead released in gasoline exhaust, cadmium and mercury, insecticides and weed killers, the industrial chemical PCB, and assorted petrochemicals, preservatives, caustic agents, and detergents contained in such commonly used household items as clothing, cosmetics, wall coverings, and cleaners. Although the medical establishment has long known that birth control pills cause a lot of yeast overgrowth, no one had yet thought of linking the condition with the invidious poisons that daily assault a woman's body.

During the normal menstrual cycle estrogen rises to a maximum when a woman is at her most fertile, causing the cervical glands to produce a sticky alkaline secretion. This raises the vaginal pH level, providing an ideal environment for vaginal infection. Menstrual flow further raises alkalinity, and during pregnancy the high level is sustained for several months. This is why birth control pills, which simulate pregnancy, invite candida to colonize at will.[3]

Antibiotics also like to make room for candida by wiping out normal, friendly bacteria while destroying their disease-causing cousins. With the good bacteria gone, the fungus steps in to take its place. Today, although they are still a godsend, antibiotics are prescribed so routinely that their targets have built up a resistance to them. To kill harmful microbes, larger and larger dosages of antibiotics have to be administered, placing a tremendous stress on the immune system while allowing candida to gain a foothold.

But candida's very best friend is sugar and other highly refined carbohydrates. Eating sweets, Dr. Crook states, is like "pouring kerosene on smoldering logs." The hungry little funguses thrive on glucose, which the body distills from the foods we eat. The more sticky sweets, cakes, pies, and junk food we eat, the more glucose we have circulating in our systems. With an average of 130 pounds annually to feed on, not to mention pounds of bleached white flour, candida is very well taken care of indeed.

Vaginal secretions normally hold a large amount of glucose, which is what gives these discharges their high alkaline quality. Under normal conditions a welcome resident called Döderlein's bacillus converts this glucose into lactic acid, thus lowering the alkalinity and preventing the fungus from colonizing. Eating too much sugar and refined carbohydrates throws this natural ecology out of whack, producing a state of clinical disease. A study conducted at the University of Alabama in the mid-1970s indicates that sugar also interferes with the ability of white blood cells to fight off bacterial assaults.[4]

In healthy persons with strong immune systems, a single candida infection would probably be dealt with promptly by the body's own bacteria-fighting antibodies. But when one considers how many women use birth control pills, take antibiotics, and indulge themselves with unhealthy foods, it's easy to see why there has been a widespread outbreak of vaginal infections in all age groups. As with hypoglycemia (see Chapter 6), the symptoms of which resemble candidiasis, the patient usually has a history of an addiction to sweets.

Because of their anatomies, men do not suffer from candida infections of the reproductive organs in the same manner as women, although suffer they do. Sexually, men are carriers more often than victims, but when the immune system has been stressed the penis, especially if uncircumcised, may break out in an inconvenient rash. That nagging case of jock itch or athlete's foot may actually be a candida infection, which is why it's so difficult to cure. Once entrenched, the fungus puts up a mighty battle to survive, calling for treatment with nystatin or a stronger medicine called Ketoconazole, which can produce side effects as uncomfortable as the disease.[5]

The organism is more democratic when it comes to the gut. Both men and women can be afflicted with irritable bowel syndrome, a particularly frustrating malady which has increased the patient load of many doctors within the last few years. The major symptoms are abdominal cramping, bloating, gassiness, and alternating constipation and diarrhea. These symptoms usually occur shortly after eating or after getting up in the morning. Normally, after the small intestine absorbs water and nutrients from food, the waste matter moves into the large intestine for elimination. In the case of irritable bowel syndrome, however, the muscular contractions that propel waste matter along the five-foot length of the colon are not properly synchronized. The bowels cramp erratically and excessively, throwing the entire process of elimination out of sync.

The medical profession has yet to solve the riddle of irritable bowel syndrome, and doctors usually advise patients to avoid emotional stress and prescribe minor tranquilizers or anticholin-

ergic drugs to reduce contractions of the large intestine. Many
people have thrown off the syndrome, however, by changing their
diets and being treated with nystatin—an indication of a candida
infestation. Refined sugary foods must be replaced with fiber-rich
fruits and vegetables and whole grain cereals that will help return
the action of the bowels to normal. By adding bulk to the stool,
fiber increases the diameter of the colon and helps prevent muscle
spasms.[6] Vitamin and mineral injections are often given to correct
deficiencies resulting from the bowels' reduced ability to absorb
these nutrients. While it has yet to be proven that sugar-fed candida
is the cause of irritated bowels, it seems it is at the very least one
of the threads that make up the total fabric of the syndrome.

To remedy these ubiquitous candida-related maladies in patients, Dr. Crook removes all sugar and refined carbohydrates from
the diet, as well as packaged and processed foods, processed and
smoked meats, coffee, tea, and alcohol. And for the few weeks of
Dr. Crook's regimen patients are not permitted fresh fruit or
vegetables with a high sugar content on the theory that these will
continue to feed the candida fungus. Because multiple symptoms
indicate that patients have developed an allergy to the yeast that has
been feasting on them, all foods containing yeast are strictly off
limits until the candida has been brought under control. These
include leavened bread, cheese, soured-milk products, mushrooms, vinegar, and any product containing malt or malt flavoring.

Patients are advised to avoid damp and dusty places, where
airborne yeasts like to live, and to minimize exposure to the
everyday chemicals found in bleach, mothballs, glues, paint,
synthetic fabrics, cosmetics, and bonded wood products. Fumes
from these items place undue demands on the immune system and
help open the door to a proliferation of yeasts. Room air filters are
also recommended to remove pollutants and yeast from rooms
patients spend the most time in.

For all their success in treating yeast infections, Doctors Truss and Crook have had to take a lot of flak from the American medical establishment. In the summer of 1986 the American Academy of Allergy and Immunology published a two-page statement declaring that their candida treatments were "speculative and unproven."[7] The academy complained that yeast therapies had not been proven in long-term clinical studies and laboratory experiments. The cures, stated the academy and others, were actually due to the "placebo effect"—that is, because the patient believes the treatment will work. Heaping accusation upon accusation, the academy dismissed, inexplicably, the anti-candida diet as being unsound. What it didn't criticize was the relationship between excessive sugar-eating and yeast infections.

The doctors have responded by letting their work speak for itself. Anecdotal evidence may not be good enough for the medical establishment, but it is more than adequate for those cured of lingering candida-related illnesses. Both doctors have impressive credentials, so it is unlikely they will be forced to abandon their treatments. Dr. Truss graduated from Cornell Medical College in New York and taught at Alabama Medical College, and Dr. Crook was educated and trained at the University of Virginia, the Pennsylvania Hospital, and Johns Hopkins. "The road to better health will not be found through more drugs, doctors, and hospitals," says Dr. Crook. "Instead, it will be discovered through better nutrition and changes in life-styles."

11

The Major Killers

"Every day you do one of two things: build health or produce disease in yourself."

—*Adelle Davis*

WHEN EPIDEMIOLOGISTS try to find out why disease rates are escalating in a given country, they always look for clues in its environment and dietary habits. In many countries, including Italy, Greece, Iceland, and Japan, the population formerly got about two-thirds of its calories from complex carbohydrates derived from grains and cereals. Since the end of World War II, as these countries became affluent, they have gradually shifted their food preferences to red meat, fats, and sugar. The rapid changeover in these countries is paralleled by rising rates of colon and breast cancer and arterial disease.[1]

The link between the Western diet and disease is obvious, even to a nonepidemiologist. These are essentially the same changes, of course, that have occurred in the United States. But how can this be? Aren't we living longer than ever before, mostly due to improved medical care?

The answer is yes, we *are* living longer than ever before, and no, it's not because of better medicines and surgeries.

While it's true that our ancestors had to fight off a heavy assault of microbes that picked many of them off before old age, those who survived lived relatively free of the diseases that bring us down today. Obesity, hypertension, diabetes, lung cancer, atherosclerotic heart disease, tooth decay, and other diseases of civilization were rare.

The forces responsible for increasing our life expectancy from about forty-nine years of age in 1900 to seventy-two today are not primarily medical, at least not in the sense of treating patients. We are living longer because of an improvement in cleanliness, because we have better housing, and because we have enough to eat. It wasn't medicine that removed tuberculosis, cholera, typhoid fever, and diarrhea from the list of major killers in the nineteenth century. It was plumbing, the creation of sewer systems, standardized garbage collection, and the sanitizing of food supplies. We saved ourselves from bacterial infection by preventing it.

Today we face a new kind of challenge: how to cope with the threats to health that accompanied the dramatic changes in our life-styles. Ever widening is the gap between how much our bodies can withstand and the demands technological society places on them. In the past, our prehistoric ancestors had plenty of evolutionary time to determine which foods were life-promoting and which were not. If someone found a nourishing food that kept him vigorous and strong, he no doubt passed on the word and others added the food to their diets. If he was wrong that became apparent over the aeons too, and the food was avoided.

We no longer have the time to progress by trial and error, however. New processed foods are being shoved into our mouths every day and it is folly to stand by and wait and see if they will produce illness decades later or result in premature death. Evolution has no time to catch up to us.

Medical science looks at this quandary from the point of view of technology. We live in a technological society, the logic goes, so we have to eat a technological diet. There can be no turning back. Any illnesses resulting from the failure of our biologies to adapt will be dealt with by technical progress in medicine. Doctors are aware that dietary factors play a critical role in heart disease, cancer, and diabetes, three of our major killers, but instead they look in vain for medical solutions that conform to our processed food system and which will not disturb the status quo.[2]

A case in point is sugar and its imitations. The voice of the medical establishment no longer addresses itself very loudly to these menaces to our physical and mental health. Its collective concern has been focused on the dangers of saturated fats and the benefits of fiber. American sugar interests are powerful and our addiction is strong; maybe it's futile to tell us to break the habit. Meanwhile, apparatus-filled operating rooms are at the ready, waiting to perform yet another heart by-pass operation and to excise another tumor.

But evolution also gave us a reasoning brain, and if we know why our ancestors didn't die from heart attacks, we should be capable of making our own wise food choices too. The keys to adding happy years to our lives are knowledge, common sense, and will power. These too are part of our evolutionary heritage.

DIABETES

Clinicians used to think that diabetes was caused by eating too much sugar, but now we know that isn't true. Not that sugar has been absolved, however. It still plays an important part in both the cause of diabetes and its treatment.

Diabetes is a failure of the body's energy regulation system. Because the pancreas can no longer secrete adequate insulin to burn glucose in the blood, the body begins to convert its fat and protein into sugar as an emergency measure. As these materials are broken down, poisonous by-products called ketones are produced, causing the diabetic to become dizzy, nauseated, and, in the final stages, comatose. The unabsorbed glucose is released by the blood and disposed of in the urine, along with many water-soluble vitamins and minerals.

Diabetes is a truly terrible disease. It sneaks up on the victim slowly, and often announces itself only after damage has been done. If not controlled by diet and, in severe cases, injections of insulin, diabetes can rupture small blood vessels in the eyes, damage the kidneys, and reduce blood flow to the feet, leading to amputation of the toes or an entire foot. Diabetes is the country's No. 4 killer and the cause of one in every three cases of blindness. The death toll may even be higher since death certificates often blame complications rather than diabetes itself.[3]

And the saddest part of the story is that diabetes, in many cases, is largely preventable. Although we inherit a predisposition to diabetes, what and how much we eat and drink throughout our early lives seems to be the determining factor.

Adult-onset diabetes is a disease of progress. It usually shows up only after the age of forty, after a lifetime of pumping ourselves full of sugar, white flour, and fats. At least 80 percent of diabetics were or are obese, and the vast majority of diabetics live in industrialized countries with the greatest sweet tooths. Refined carbohydrates, coffee, nicotine, alcohol, and stress all cause the adrenal glands to work overtime, and the overstimulation causes the pancreas to literally wear out. Experiments have shown that rats bred to be genetically susceptible to diabetes do not develop the disease unless they are overfed. The same connection was observed in Europe during World War II: the incidence of diabetes declined dramatically when shortages substantially reduced the availability of sugar and other rich foods.[4]

So far, medical science has not been able to come up with a cure, and the best it can do is administer insulin. A Canadian, Dr.

Frederick Banting, and a Scot, John J.R. Macleod, discovered this imperfect alternative and were awarded a Nobel Prize in 1923. Drug companies, eager to exploit a captive market of a million or so diabetics, a market that was certain to grow, hailed insulin as one of the first miracles of modern medical science. But as William Dufty points out in his *Sugar Blues,* Dr. Banting later "tried to tell us that his discovery was merely a palliative, not a cure, and that the way to prevent diabetes was to cut down on dangerous sugar binging."

"In the U.S. the incidence of diabetes has increased proportionately with the per capita consumption of sugar," Dr. Banting pointed out many years after his discovery.

"In the heating and recrystallization of the natural sugarcane, something is altered which leaves the refined products a dangerous foodstuff."[5]

CANCER

No word in the English language is more dreaded than *cancer.* We know it is is the second greatest killer among diseases and wonder if we will be the one in four who will be stricken this year. There are seldom clear and obvious warnings. There are no physical examinations that will rule out the possibility we have it. There are no absolute cures.

It's not a losing battle, however. We can fight back by removing harmful substances from our diet and environment and thereby increase the odds in our favor. Like diabetes, most cancers appear in people over forty. A tumor takes many years to develop. Irritated for years and lacking in the elements they need, cells lose their natural controls and begin to multiply out of control. Other organs cannot do their proper work, and pieces of cancer tissue may break off and, carried by the blood or lymph system, start growing in new parts of the body.

Many cancers seem to originate in response to industrial and environmental pollutants, but others, like breast cancer and colon cancer, have been shown to be related to diet. Victims of breast cancer, the leading killer of women, are, on average, heavy consumers of fats and sugar. In addition, many of these women are overweight, some to the point of obesity, from eating an excess of these foods. Too much extra body fat, studies indicate, stimulates female hormones and enhances the growth of cancers that have already formed.[6]

What has been conspicuously lacking in the diets of women with breast cancer is fiber, B complex vitamins, vitamin A, and essential minerals that the immune system must have to work properly. Japanese women, for example, eat much more fiber than we do and significantly less sugar and fat. As a result, breast cancer is relatively uncommon there. But when Japanese women emigrate to the United States (as shown by a number of "war brides" brought home by GIs after World War II and the Korean War), and adopt the American diet, their breast cancer rate begins to rise to the level of American women.[7]

To reduce your risk of cancer (and heart disease as well) the National Research Council recommends reducing fat to no more than 30 percent of calorie intake (we are currently consuming about 37 to 50 percent), or, better yet, cutting your intake of fats and oils in half. The average American should consume about 65 percent more whole grains than he or she does at present, and legumes (beans) by more than 75 percent.

Colon cancer often follows years of constipation. In a very real sense, constipation is a self-induced condition. The victim generally gets very little exercise and eats highly refined foods that contain little bulk—which might be the definition of a couch potato television addict. The feces become hardened and difficult to pass because they are unable to absorb water. The waste matter then has to remain in the large intestine for a longer than normal period, allowing the colon to absorb even more water, as well as many soluble poisons.

This gives bacteria that live in the intestinal track ample time to convert these bilious body wastes into deoxycholic acid, a known cancer-causing agent. Ample fiber in the diet moves wastes along faster, so there is little time for this chemical reaction to occur. The benefits of a low-sugar, low-fat, high-fiber diet can be seen in Seventh Day Adventists who live in the United States. Their vegetarian, grain-based diet has largely prevented them from developing colon cancer. And in Africa and India, where fiber intake is high, bowel diseases are practically nonexistent. The stool of an African native passes through his body in from thirty to thirty-five hours; the stool of the average young American takes about three days to make the journey.[8]

ATHEROSCLEROSIS

Wherever people live on a diet high in sugar, white flour, and saturated animal fats, heart disease is certain to follow. Over time, the diet produces an excess of yellowish gunk and deposits it in the arteries. The gunk, called cholesterol, continues to accumulate, narrowing these pathways to the heart and undermining their flexibility. One day, before you know it, bingo! You've got atherosclerosis and are a candidate for a by-pass operation.

In 1970 nearly a million people died of cardiovascular disease. Today that figure is down to less than 600,000. Experts attribute this improved mortality rate to that fact that many of us have cut down on meat, eggs, and cigarettes, are drinking less alcohol, and are relaxing and exercising more.[9] We are also being diagnosed earlier, and, in addition, there are new drugs available to dilate blood vessels and help the blood get through. But even though the death rate has been reduced, heart disease remains the No. 1 killer, so we must be doing something wrong.

Maybe it's because taking saturated fats out of the diet is not the entire answer. Refined carbohydrates, especially sugar, have been shown to act in conjunction with saturated fats to increase triglycerides (fatty substances) in the blood. And refined carbohydrates and saturated fats pretty much describe the American diet. Take a typical fast food meal, for example: a hamburger (saturated fat and sugar and refined white flour in the bun, sugar in the sauce and pickle); a cola drink (sugar) or a milkshake (hydrogenated fat, a little milk fat and sugar); French fries (starch, sugar in the ketchup).

Can it be that sugar is more to blame for arterial degeneration than saturated fats? In the last hundred years, the consumption of saturated fat has increased by only about 20 percent. The consumption of sugar, other sweeteners, and refined carbohydrates has increased by a mind-boggling 700 percent.[10]

Back in the 1970s, Dr. John Yudkin, professor of nutrition and dietetics at the University of London, brought this connection to light. His studies showed that even when a person ate only four ounces of sugar a day, or half as much as we presently eat, that person faced more than five times the normal risk of developing heart disease. Yudkin maintained, quite accurately, that sugar creates cravings that lead to overeating. When an individual eats more than he needs, triglycerides increase.[11] Although the medical establishment largely ignored Yudkin's research and relegated it to a dusty back room, newer research indicates how correct he was.

Again, insulin, that hormone so put upon by sugar, makes an appearance. In a valiant attempt to get rid of the excess sugar, it instructs the body to turn it into triglycerides and fatty acids. In a study conducted by the Department of Agriculture at its Beltsville, Maryland, nutrition laboratory, a group of volunteers were placed on a six-week diet. Half were given a daily diet consisting of 30 percent sugar, and the other half were given 30 percent more whole grains. At the end of the experiment the heavily sugared group had nearly a third more fat in their blood than the group that had eaten the cereals. Sugar, it was found in another study, may also enhance the effects of salt in increasing blood pressure.[12]

And the saturated fats connection doesn't hold when one considers traditional Eskimos and other northern peoples who consume lots of animal fats. Their incidence of heart disease is drastically lower than that of their more civilized urban neighbors to the south.

The Centers for Disease Control estimates that over twenty million people are carbohydrate-sensitive, which means they have an inherited tendency to clog their arteries with cholesterol when they eat sugar. It's an interesting statistic. But in the quantities we Americans consume sugar, we have probably all become carbohydrate-sensitive.

12

Natural Foods or Nutritional Traps?

"Nature uses as little as possible of anything."
—*Johannes Kepler*

IN THE STILL budding interest in better health, many people are turning to foods variously termed "natural," "organic," or "health foods." These terms are reassuring to shoppers confused by the misinformation and infobabble that still surround nutrition issues. In most cases, however, they're merely catchphrases employed by processed food manufacturers to lure the health-conscious into the fold.

"Lite" or "light" is the latest misnomer employed by the food industry to entice the calorie- and health-conscious consumer. At present there are over 700 products on the market that display these words on their labels. While they suggest that a product is lower in sugar and fat calories, what they mean is often something quite to the contrary. The Food and Drug Administration and the U.S. Department of Agriculture, the government agencies that regulate the boundaries of product labeling, have been remarkably lax in protecting the consumer against this increasingly common deception.[1]

Under USDA regulations, the term applies only to processed meats, while the FDA states that a "lite" product must have at least one-third fewer calories than the regular product. With these exceptions, manufacturers are free to label high-calorie products as "lite" simply because they are lighter in color, flavor, or texture. Investigators of the Public Voice for Food and Health Policy, a Washington, D.C., based consumer advocacy group, found that some "lite" soups actually were higher in calories than the regular product. Similarly, many "light" oils, especially olive oils, were found to contain the same amount of fat as the regular brands. Another subterfuge is to call a product "lite" based on an unrealistic serving size recommended on the package. Few of us could probably restrict ourselves to the one-ounce serving of "lite" and "natural" potato chips that have recently appeared on supermarket shelves.

Coming up with legal definitions of "natural" and "health food" probably would be impossible. And "organic" in its strictest sense merely means food derived from plants or animals. A few states have laws on the books defining "organic," but these vary widely, and not even the Federal Trade Commission can decide what the word means. What we think we're getting when we buy foods so labeled is another matter. The common assumption is that they are grown without chemical pesticides and fertilizers, antibiotics and hormones, and were delivered to the store with no preservatives, artificial colorings, and flavorings—and no added sugar.

In fact, there is no guarantee that you will not get any or all of the above when you buy a "natural" product. And of all the chemicals added to food, none is more ubiquitous than refined white sugar and high fructose corn syrup, its fraternal twin. The marketing assumption is—and sales figures, unfortunately, bear this out—that Americans do not want to take their nutrition straight. Natural, relatively unprocessed foods that gained their reputations because of their health-promoting qualities are routinely sweetened up. Many of us now actually like yogurt, oatmeal, and granola, and we're eating more salads and tofu than ever. But what we're getting for our money may not be what we expected.

YOGURT

Yogurt may not prolong life, as many formerly believed, but in its natural state it is about as nutritious a food as you can get. Yogurt is milk—generally cow's milk—which is curdled by the action of two strains of bacteria. Eight ounces supplies from 20 percent to 25 percent of your daily protein requirement and gives you 300 to 400 milligrams of calcium. There's also a goodly supply of riboflavin, phosphorus, and potassium.

The best yogurt, considering how much fat Americans get in other foods, is low-fat yogurt made from skim milk with added milk solids. The calorie count is only 90 to 110 and you'll get up to 450 milligrams of calcium. Whole milk brings the calorie count up to 140 to 210 and lowers the calcium level to 275 to 400. Whole milk yogurt, at about 320 milligrams per 8-ounce glass, also has seven times the cholesterol.

Yogurt is especially beneficial for kids and adults whose systems can't tolerate milk. The bacteria convert most of the lactose (milk sugar) into lactic acid, which is what gives yogurt its tang. Yogurt can also be helpful in restoring a healthy balance of microbes that live in your gastrointestinal system, especially after treatment with antibiotics or when you've had a yeast-infection—another sugar-related illness (see Chapter 10).

Although still promoted as a health food, yogurt has undergone a remarkable transformation to make it more palatable to Americans. The Middle Easterners and Bulgarians who have been making yogurt for years (and eat as much as six pounds a day) probably wouldn't recognize the gussied-up products in our refrigerators. It may sound encouraging that since 1965 our consumption of yogurt has gone up about ten times (to about three and a half pounds per person per year[2]), but the concoctions on the market are not quite yogurt. They are laced with sugar syrups and made to resemble ice cream to mask the tart flavor of fermented milk for the majority of us who will eat only sweet things.

Plain yogurt has no extra calories, but vanilla, lemon, and coffee flavors contain the equivalent of three and a half teaspoons of sugar. Add some gooey berry or cherry jam, and you'll get up to seven teaspoons of sugar. The jam in Swiss- and French-style yogurts is premixed and held in place by a solidifying agent such as gelatin, and the newer products resemble puddings in consistency because of added stabilizers and preservatives. Frozen low-fat yogurt may be better for you than ice cream from a cholesterol point of view, but it contains just as much sugar as ice cream. What these additions do is replace some of yogurt's nutritional value and lower the amount of calcium by from 50 to 100 milligrams.[3]

Recently introduced are products that sound and look like yogurt but are actually extra-sweet synthetic puddings that are a solidified version of nondairy creamer. For those put off by yogurt's tartness, kefir, a related fermented-milk product, is available in many health food stores. Made from a different strain of bacteria, this age-old food gets its sweetness from the milk itself.

OATS

Oats are good for you because they are one of the few cereals that retain the whole grain and *all* of their fiber when converted into hot cereal. Eaten with milk, oatmeal is a complete protein and the least expensive breakfast you can buy. It's a good source of calcium, the B vitamins, inositol, and a number of trace minerals. The English and Irish prefer their oats steel-cut, which is a good idea because fewer nutrients are lost to the high heat oats are submitted to before being rolled.[4]

Oat bran, which is the outer layer of oat grain, offers even more fiber than the whole grain but isn't as tasty. (A one-ounce serving of oat bran has 2.2 grams of fiber versus 1.5 grams in oatmeal.)

Oat bran came out of the shadow of its more familiar parent in 1987 after a study at Northwestern University Medical School showed that sixty-nine volunteers who ate thirty-nine grams of oat bran every day for a month and a half reduced their cholesterol count by 3 percent. Another study, at the University of Kentucky, gave ten volunteers a hundred grams of oat bran a day and reduced their cholesterol count by 19 percent in only twenty-one days.[5] Articles appeared in medical journals and popular magazines, and when Robert E. Kowalski recommended oat bran in his best-selling *The 8-Week Cholesterol Cure,* the race was on. The food industry lost no time in coopting the soluble fiber and sprinkling it into a variety of high-calorie products. Banners appeared on boxes of some sweetened breakfast cereals, cookies, potato chips, and other junk foods pointing out, by implication, that because they contained minuscule amounts of oat bran they were now more nutritious.

But what the much-heralded studies showed was that oat bran has to be in the system every day to lower cholesterol. And the amount required—a hundred grams of bran—means that you must eat one-third of a cup twice a day. No muffin, cookie, or bread approaches that level, and some of those highest in oat bran are also highest in sweeteners.

Quaker, the leading producer of oats and oat bran in the United States, is well aware of what people really want, as evidenced by its Fruit & Cream line. Quaker's Strawberries & Cream instant oatmeal, for example, is loaded with artery-clogging coconut oil, red dye, and sulfites. The strawberries inside the box are apple pieces doused with sugar, artificial flavoring, dye, and strawberry solids from concentrate.

THE SALAD BAR

When it first appeared in restaurants and supermarkets back in the 1970s, the salad bar offered a commendable selection of raw vegetables and fruit. Today it is a caricature of its former self and more closely resembles a delicatessen counter. Like yogurt before it, the salad bar has tripped down the primrose path, into adulteration with fat, sugar, and salt. Once the sweetheart of health professionals, it has become a nutritional minefield that must be treaded carefully.[6]

A close inspection of a typical salad bar will reveal that the bad now outnumbers the good. For every bowl of unadorned carrot or green pepper slices, there are matching bowls of shredded carrots swimming in a mayonnaise sauce and sweet and sour pickles oozing syrup. Broccoli isn't considered palatable unless tossed into a cold pasta salad with a sweet dressing to heighten its chilled flavors. And shredded cabbage moves faster when mixed into a large mold of orange-flavored Jell-O. Luckily for us, most sliced fruits on the counter are left unadorned.

In adding customer appeal to the salad bar, restaurant and supermarket owners have diluted the nutritional worth of raw vegetables. If the greens and tomatoes aren't already dripping with a creamy dressing—the preferred variety—we pour on an ample amount ourselves. According to the Department of Agriculture's National Food Review, we ate more salads in 1987 than we did in 1985; but during that period we also ate more sugar, fats, and oil—the same ingredients that have polluted the salad bar.

You can still put together a nutritious salad at a salad bar, but if you choose the prepared items don't delude yourself that you are eating healthily. You may as well break down and have a slice of pizza. You'll get a better nutritional bargain.

GRANOLA

Revived in the 1960s, this turn-of-the-century whole grain cereal has found a permanent place on supermarket and health food store shelves. Granolas are high in vitamins, minerals, amino acids, and fiber since they are comprised of rolled oats, wheat germ, and other grains, and nuts, seeds, and dried fruit. This is the way granola was originally served by Dr. John Harvey Kellogg and C.W. Post (who both claimed to have invented it) at their health clinics in the 1890s.[7] Today's granola, however, is spiced with coconut shreds and sprayed with liquid brown sugar on the assembly line. The coconut, which is usually sweetened, adds measurably to the oils found in the nuts and seeds, and the overall calorie count is considerable. Half a cup of granola in the bowl may seem like a puny breakfast, but it contains about 250 calories. Health food brands are usually sweetened with honey or molasses, which make not a whit of difference.

TOFU

Sometimes referred to as "the meat that grows on trees," tofu is actually a curd made from fermented soybeans. While its protein is not equivalent to that of meat or fish, tofu is superior to other vegetable proteins and low in carbohydrates but rich in vitamins and minerals. The Chinese and Japanese have been eating it for centuries,[8] but it never quite took off when it arrived in the United

States. That is, not until it was blended with sugars, tempered with chemicals, whipped into a froth, frozen, and called Tofutti. This "diet" dessert, pitched to cholesterol watchers, quickly found its niche in the marketplace. Many Tofutti fanciers also believe the product is low in calories: It is not. Maple walnut Tofutti, for instance, contains 230 calories per half-cup serving, as opposed to the 150 calories of ordinary supermarket ice cream.[9] Only the "lite" variety has fewer calories, but this dessert is so insubstantial on the tongue that it may well drive dieting ice cream fanciers back to the real thing. What Tofutti has going for it is that it is dairy-free (a plus for the lactose-intolerant) and contains no fat (although some brands of frozen tofu do). But it is also heavily sugared and has no calcium and few of the other benefits of real tofu.

"Natural" foods, as you can see, aren't necessarily what manufacturers say they are. One day, perhaps, when consumers decide to flex their muscle, the FTC will put into effect its 1978 definition of "natural." The word, said the commission, should refer only to foods that are "minimally processed." These products should contain no synthetic additives or flavor or color additives whether artificial or natural. For its part, the Food and Drug Administration merely forbids manufacturers from labeling an entire product "natural" if it contains any artificial ingredients. That's as far as it goes. Food processors can easily squeeze through this loophole by making the claim about only a part of their product.

Thus, beverage manufacturers can say their drinks have "100% natural flavors," even though they contain only 10 percent real juice. The remainder is water, sugar and/or corn sweetener, and preservatives. Cheesemakers are permitted to label their factory-produced cheddars and Swisses as "natural" to distinguish them from process cheese, even though most contain potassium sorbate and calcium chloride as preservatives. And "natural" beers have never seen the inside of a traditional brewing vat. Beer is made from barley and sugar, natural enough, then injected with carbon dioxide and tannic acid added to keep it from going flat.

But perhaps the most surprising claim of all comes from the Sugar Association. In a series of print ads that have been running since 1986, the Association claims that its product is "100% Natural . . . and perfectly safe."

13

Addiction Times Two

"First you take a drink, then the drink takes a drink, then the drink takes you."

—*F. Scott Fitzgerald*

In 1987 alcohol killed about 100,000 people—more than twenty-five times as many as those terminated by crack, heroin, and all other illegal drugs combined.[1] It seems likely that this figure, based on a government tally of death certificates, is on the low side. Other surveys indicate many families are too embarrassed to tell the truth and list other causes on death certificates. Easier to determine are the number of traffic fatalities caused by alcohol abuse. According to U.S. Surgeon General C. Everett Koop, there is one alcohol-related death on the nation's highways every twenty-two minutes. In addition, more than two million drivers are arrested every year for driving under the influence of alcohol.

According to a recent Gallup Poll, one in four families has a member with a drinking problem—the highest incidence in nearly half a century. Government statisticians estimate there are about 10.6 million alcoholics in the United States—a figure that beats all previous records. About seven million more are problem drinkers, mostly young men, who often go on troublemaking binges.[2]

Imbibed only occasionally and in moderation, alcohol is no more harmful than an occasional teaspoon of sugar in the majority of users. The trouble is that the line between social drinking and

121

drinking to the point of intoxication is easily blurred. Frequent drinkers may find themselves sliding into the abyss of alcoholism without being aware of their fall. Like its parent—sugar—alcohol is a crafty seducer. It offers the alcoholic a Mephistophelian bargain of illusory pleasure in return for the victim's mental and physical health.

By definition, alcoholism is an illness characterized by an inability to stay away from alcohol or to control the amount consumed. Alcoholics can't get through the day without their favorite mood-enhancers. They rationalize away their addiction by claiming they need "a lift," "something to calm my nerves," or "a little something to help me sleep."

If this diagnosis and these rationalizations sound familiar, that's because alcoholism and sugar addiction are remarkably alike. Both addicts obsessively drink and eat their favorite poisons and, as a result, both suffer the same nutritional defects. Evidence suggests the two addictions may in actuality be one and the same.

No one can dispute that psychological influences may point an individual in the direction of alcoholism, or that hereditary predisposition plays a part in the disease, but not everyone under severe stress or whose parent was a heavy drinker becomes an alcohol abuser. Often, what precipitates an alcohol problem is a sugar problem. Researchers have long noted that heavy drinkers have well-developed sweet tooths which can become ravenous when they attempt to give up alcohol. What's wrong with our current mode of diagnosis was pointed out back in 1971 (and nothing has since changed) by Dr. Roger Williams.[3] The medical establishment has confused cause with effect: malnutrition of the brain cells doesn't only result from alcoholism, it causes it.

Dr. Williams's conclusions were verified by an experiment at Linda Loma University in California, which showed that a sugary diet can create alcoholics.

The experiment involved thirty rats, an animal which, like it or not, is similar in biological response to human beings. The rats were divided into three groups of ten each. One group was fed a diet high in white sugar and bleached flour, and low in protein, vitamins, and minerals. The second group got the same highly refined diet along with vitamin and mineral supplements. The third group ate properly balanced human meals. None of the rats were stressed or otherwise abused.

Several weeks later, researchers gave the rats a choice between water and a solution of 10 percent alcohol. Those who had been fed the nutritionally empty diet showed a marked preference for the alcohol-laced water, and by the end of the experiment they were drinking it almost exclusively. Rats on the fortified junk diet drank the alcohol only about a third as much, while those who had eaten well retained their preference for water. Moreover, when sugar was added to the alcohol solution consumed by several of the drunken rodents, these became the most avid boozers of all. At the end of the experiment sixteen weeks later, the heavy drinkers were given a balanced diet and nearly all lost their taste for alcohol.[4]

The Linda Loma researchers' inescapable conclusion was that alcoholism is, in large measure, a metabolic disorder that can be corrected by staying away from the wrong foods and eating the right ones. As the late Carlton Fredericks pointed out, ''The alcoholic substitutes alcohol for food; the sugarholic substitutes sugar for food.''

Approximately 90 percent of diagnosed alcoholics suffer from low blood sugar, many to the point of hypoglycemia (see Chapter 6), which is commonly blamed on the alcohol consumed. But the problem has probably been simmering for years, long before alcohol entered the picture. Alcoholics are also known to be heavy drinkers of coffee and cola drinks, whose caffeine exacerbates the pancreas's fatigue by constantly attempting to adjust the level of sugar in the blood. Alcoholics also tend to smoke, calling forth another stimulant, nicotine, to further throw the metabolism out of kilter.

Cigarettes, of course, are as addictive as alcohol, if not more so. That the two frequently go hand in hand isn't surprising since sugar plays a part in the manufacture of both substances. Smokers would no doubt be surprised if you told them they were smoking sugar, but indeed they are. The tobacco in American cigarettes, cigars, and pipe tobacco is treated with sugar to improve flavor and burning quality. The amount varies from 10 to 20 percent according to the type of tobacco. Chewing tobacco, which has become a popular alternative to smoking, often contains considerably more.[5] What part burning sugar may play in the development of lung cancer has yet to be investigated.

Since alcohol gives an even quicker blood sugar rise than sugar, going from sugar to alcohol is for many a natural progression. Alcohol is the ultimate refined carbohydrate. The stimulus to drink is usually social, to share a communal glass of cheer with friends, relatives, and colleagues. Before long, the social drinker is experiencing a rapid blood sugar rise with each cocktail. Since alcohol is absorbed into the body even faster than sugar, habitual drinking can create a craving even greater than sugar craving.

The origin of alcohol goes back at least two million years, when man probably chanced on it accidentally. The first brew may have been tree sap that had fermented in a hollow branch. Spirits have been part of our history ever since, but it wasn't until the arrival of refined sugar that drinking became widespread. Alcohol is made by microscopic plants called yeasts, which will spontaneously attack the sugar in any solution. Given the right temperature, they change the sugar into a colorless liquid called alcohol, or, more precisely, ethyl alcohol, the kind we drink. The process is called fermentation.

The best raw materials for making alcohol are sugary ones, such as sugarcane (rum), fruit (brandy), and honey (mead), or starchy substances, such as rye (whiskey), corn (bourbon), potatoes (vodka), and rice (sake). In the past, supply was dictated by the availability of crops harvested in a given area. When white sugar became widely available, it was commonly added to the fermentation process to vastly increase alcohol yields.

In Russia, a country that consumes even more alcohol than the United States, authorities have inaugurated a not-very-popular anti-alcohol campaign. One of their first moves was to ration sugar in an attempt to control a prospering moonshine industry. To a sugar-loving society, where heavily sweetened tea, homemade cakes, and sugar jams are staples of hospitality, this was very bad news indeed. But without rationing, the Soviet government would have had to lay out about $1 billion of scarce foreign currency to import enough sugar to compensate for stocks depleted by distillers of illegal alcohol, called samogen. Russian citizens, an authority commented, "will have to choose between samogen and their sweet tooth."[6]

In the United States, however, there is plenty of sugar and alcohol to go around. The two, in fact, are often combined to satisfy the sugar hunger of a new generation of American drinkers. The drink of choice in bars and restaurants frequented by people in their twenties is usually a technicolored one. Current favorites are blueberry daiquiris and blue margaritas, green Midori melon balls, and pinkish-orange woo-woos, concocted of vodka, cranberry juice (heavily sweetened), and peach schnapps (also heavily sweetened).

Many of these young drinkers got their training from wine coolers, a carbonated, wine-based beverage introduced in the early 1980s. Bottled to resemble soda pop, they usually omit the word "wine" on labels in favor of a connotation more appealing to adolescents: Berry Cooler, White Mountain, Sun Country, and the like. They are marketed like soft drinks on television commercials with cartoons and animals to show how much fun they are to drink. The spirits industry has spent more dollars advertising these beverages than on any other alcoholic drink.[7]

Beset by declining alcohol consumption and stiffer regulations, the industry decided to pitch coolers to young people, the majority of whom had rejected the traditional drinks of their elders as being bitter and medicinal-tasting. The plan apparently was that young drinkers would eventually graduate from coolers to more expensive wines and liquors. The repackaging of inferior products with sugar had previously worked wonders in the food industry, so why not try it with alcohol? The industry's gamble paid off handsomely, for by 1986 retail sales of coolers had reached $1.6 billion. Although sales slackened the following year,[8] the trend was partially offset by sales of wine and distilled spirits. As predicted, the sweet bubbly drinks seemed to have led to a desire for the hard stuff. It was a virtual replay, on a mass scale, of the Linda Loma experiment.

Meanwhile, the cooler habit has passed to a generation of Americans who shouldn't be drinking them at all. A 1987 survey released by the Metropolitan Life Insurance Company showed that by age twelve, 40 percent of American youngsters have sampled wine coolers. Since the weight of a twelve-year-old averages about 70 pounds, the alcohol content of a wine cooler would have considerably more impact than on a 150-pound adult.

Even though every state but Wyoming has raised its minimum drinking age to twenty-one, surveys indicate there has been little slowdown in teenage drinking habits. The No. 1 favorite alcoholic beverage among teenagers is beer, which isn't surprising since by age eighteen they have viewed an estimated 100,000 beer commercials.[9] High school and college students are now prime targets of alcoholic beverage manufacturers, who peddle their products at industry-sponsored rock concerts and sporting events. The Surgeon General places much of the blame for the increasing number of school-age drinkers on these commercial tie-ins. Dr. Koop threw down the gauntlet in the spring of 1989 by pointing an angry finger at beer, wine, and liquor companies. "Certain advertising and marketing practices for alcoholic beverages," accused Dr. Koop, "direct the wrong messages to college students and other youths who are clearly under the legal drinking age." Dr. Koop's proposal that all such advertising be banned was met with angry protests from the industry—a reaction similar to the outrage of crack dealers who protest innocence when chased from a school corner.

Some teenagers pick up the alcohol habit at home, however, from parents who drink or are relieved that their children are drinking alcohol rather than taking drugs. But alcohol is the most widely abused drug of all: it is socially approved and available everywhere. As one researcher at Emory University's Addiction Disorder Program pointed out, using alcohol in place of drugs is "like switching seats on the *Titanic*."

Teenagers and adults drink for the same reason. It's the sweetness that gets many teenagers hooked, but ultimately it's not the taste they are after, but the sweet afterglow. The euphoric effect is similar to the effect of a barbiturate, both of which depress certain parts of the brain. Contrary to popular supposition, alcohol is not a stimulant. It slows down brain centers that control behavior and judgment. When we are in our cups we become less inhibited, less self-critical, and our anxieties, tensions, and feelings of inadequacy disappear. Used in moderation, alcohol can foster an atmosphere of conviviality and good will. But alcohol is an unreliable drug. While some people may behave affectionately and garrulously, others may become combative and physically violent.

Alcohol is also a short-acting drug, which means that a sequence of drinks is required to sustain the desired effect.

When taken in excess, we stagger, slur our words, and act with even less restraint. In a word, we are drunk. Brain centers that control reflex actions and muscular movements are seriously impaired. The next morning we may not recall what took place the night before, but there is a hangover to remind us.

A hangover, of course, is a withdrawal symptom—the body's reaction to a systemic poisoning. Over time, heavy consumption of alcohol can lead to cirrhosis of the liver, a cell-destroying, silent disease that rarely shows itself until the damage is too far-gone to be treated. Alcohol-soaked brain cells wither away, leading to permanent damage of the brain and nervous system. Blood pressure increases, resulting in hypertension. The stomach lining is irritated, impairing its ability to process food. The risk of cancer is increased.[10] For pregnant women the hazards are doubled, since drinking during pregnancy can damage the fetus.

After years of foot-dragging, the U.S. Bureau of Alcohol, Tobacco and Firearms, which regulates these industries, finally took a tiny step to counteract the spirit world's mammoth advertising campaigns. And tiny is the word for it. As of November 18, 1989, all imported or domestic alcoholic beverages must bear a warning label, either on the front, side, or back of the container. Finding it may be difficult because few people look on the back of a bottle. But seeing it is harder. The BATF decreed that the labeling need only be one millimeter high on containers less than eight ounces. For 8-ounce sizes it need be only two millimeters high. In the smaller size the message reads as follows:

GOVERNMENT WARNING: 1. According to the Surgeon General, women should not drink alcoholic beverages during pregnancy because of the risk of birth defects. 2. Consumption of alcoholic beverages impairs your ability to drive a car or operate machinery, and may cause health problems.

Getting alcohol out of America's system requires a herculean effort, not a feeble gesture. Many of us live our lives in a progressive sequence of addictions: from sugar to caffeine and nicotine to alcohol. Illegal drugs are but a short step away. And when we give up one, we usually retain the others. Social scientists have even coined a new term to describe America's multiple addictions. We have become a nation of "poly-addicts."[11]

14

The Truth About Artificial Sweeteners

"There is no real evidence that artificial sweeteners help people to lose weight."
                                                —*Michael F. Jacobson*

SATISFYING our sweet tooth without the calories has become an American way of life. We're determined to have our cake and eat it too—and without gaining an ounce. Sugar surrogates, merchandisers tell us, keeping up the ballyhoo, are wonders of the technological age. They are tasty, innocuous, nondamaging to the teeth, and will keep us trim, fit, and happy. Swept under the rug is the evidence that, with the exception of a desired sweet taste, they are as dangerous to our well-being as sugar. Moreover, despite the widespread use of artificial sweeteners during the last three decades, Americans are getting fatter than ever and sales of sugar continue to soar.

SACCHARIN

Artificial sweeteners arrived by accident in 1879, when a German chemist named Constantin Fahlberg, working in a laboratory at Johns Hopkins University, touched his fingers to his mouth and discovered they tasted intensely sweet. Fahlberg had been working with coal tar, from which a number of dyes, scents, colorings, preservatives, and solvents had recently been synthesized. Repeating the experiment that had produced the illusory sensation, Fahlberg synthesized a white, crystalline powder that came to be known as saccharin,[1] after the Sanskrit root word meaning "sugar."

Because it is so sweet, a saccharin pill the size of a large pinhead is enough to sweeten a cup of coffee. Cheaper and much less bulky to handle than sugar, saccharin was given a grand welcome by the recently arrived food processing industry, looking for ways to increase profits. Before long saccharin was replacing sugar in bakery products, soft drinks, canned fruit and milk, and candies. Since ingredient labeling was not yet required by law, consumers had no way of knowing they were getting an inexpensive synthetic rather than the real thing—sugar.[2]

In the early 1900s, the growing practice of adding chemicals to food to color and flavor them, and to add shelf life, spawned the nation's first consumer movement. As a result, the Pure Food Act of 1906 was passed, prohibiting the addition of saccharin to food products in place of sugar. The chemical, consumer advocates successfully argued, deceived the public and lacked food value. Worse, its prolonged use could damage the kidneys and cause disease.

Reports of the adverse effects of saccharin on the human body had previously been circulated in the United States from France and Germany, which banned its use in food and drink. But when World War I cut off much of America's sugar supply, the ban was lifted, and saccharin has been with us ever since.

Literally hundreds of papers have been written about the damage done by saccharin. A major study by the Food and Drug Administration in 1951 linked it to cancer. And in 1969, another study by Dr. George T. Bryan, a noted cancer researcher, found that large doses of saccharin produced bladder cancer in laboratory mice. The evidence that saccharin is a carcinogen was inconclusive, however, until a 1977 study in Canada proved it without a doubt. Test animals were isolated from other factors, and only pure saccharin was used to eliminate possible contaminants. The control groups all showed an increased incidence of bladder cancer.[3] This study prompted the FDA to ban saccharin, a ruling that has been on hold ever since. Meanwhile, saccharin remains on the FDA's priority list as a possible cause of birth defects, reproductive problems, and less obvious "subacute" effects.

Research continues to go on in other countries, however. In 1983, Japanese clinicians found that saccharin can also enhance the action of other carcinogens entering the urinary tract.[4] Thus, in addition to the possibility of causing cancer itself, saccharin may be a co-carcinogen working in tandem with other risky substances like aspartame. As consumer advocate Michael F. Jacobson has pointed out, "Because cancer takes ten to twenty years to develop in humans, we do not know yet whether we shall be witnessing a cancer epidemic among those who ate diet foods."[5]

CYCLAMATE

Although it is sweet and convenient, saccharin has certain disadvantages. It leaves a somewhat bitter aftertaste when used in beverages, and it loses sweetness under the prolonged heat required by cooking, baking, and canning. So when a new compound without these drawbacks came on the market, it quickly became the nonnutritive sweetener of choice. Also derived from coal tar, cyclamate was discovered by accident in 1937, by a University of Illinois graduate student. There are two cyclamates—sodium cyclamate and calcium cyclamate, the latter for those on low-sodium diets. They are thirty times sweeter than sugar and taste more like it than saccharin does.[6]

Originally, saccharin and cyclamate were approved for use by the FDA for diabetics and others who could not tolerate sugar, and such products had to be clearly labeled: "nonnutritive, artificial sweetener which should be used only by persons who must restrict their intake of ordinary sweets." But cyclamate appeared on the market just as Americans realized they were gaining weight, so products containing cyclamate aimed their big advertising guns at those who were trying to slim down. Thus, the original warning labels were tempered to "by persons who desire . . . ," "recommended for . . . ," "nonnutritive," and, finally, the magic words "no calories."

As a rule, the formula for so-called diet food and beverages was one part saccharin to ten parts cyclamate, with each contributing about one-half of the sweetening power. By 1965 an estimated 170 million people were binging on cyclamate in every possible form: in a granulated product that resembles table sugar, in liquid drops, and in soft drinks, fruit drinks, ice cream, puddings, candy, cookies, jellies, jams, breakfast cereals, canned soups, "900-calorie" meals, salad dressings, and bread. Within ten years—from 1955 to 1965—Americans had gone from 250,000 pounds of artificial sweeteners to over 20 million pounds annually.

As consumption rose, of course, the total amount of artificial sweeteners eaten by a single individual rose to substantial proportions, causing the FDA to question the safety of cyclamate. Rumors had been circulating for years about the harm done by the endemic use of this sweetener. But the FDA had previously tested cyclamate on the basis that not much of it would be used by any one person, and now it was being consumed daily by nearly everyone. Coming on the heels of the thalidomide tragedy, these rumors sparked a number of new tests by the FDA and other research laboratories.[7]

In 1962 the FDA cautioned that "the question of the safety of cyclamate for all classes of people is not settled." The statement seemed to be calling for, at the very least, a restriction on cyclamate, but instead the FDA expanded its use to new groups of food. Meanwhile, independent medical evidence accumulated: test animals had delivered deformed fetuses, others had produced offspring with low birth weight, and many had shown signs of kidney, liver, and bone marrow damage. In 1966 Japanese researchers discovered that some people's bodies convert the sweetener into CHA, a chemical commonly used as a rust inhibitor in paint products.

The Japanese findings were duplicated in a test conducted by the Albany Medical College, in New York, in a three-month trial with thirty-two prison inmates. Seventeen of them converted cyclamate to CHA and nine developed severe diarrhea. Others showed an elevated level of iodine, which is a symptom of hyperthyroidism.

Then, in 1969, the FDA's Dr. Jacqueline Verrett appeared on NBC television advising pregnant women not to use cyclamates. Her tests had revealed that 15 percent of chicken embryos fed normal amounts of cyclamate were born deformed. The telecast lit up FDA switchboards, and a month later the Secretary of Health, Education and Welfare banned the chemical by removing it from the GRAS (Generally Regarded as Safe) list of food and drug additives. Thus, nineteen years after its introduction, this hazardous chemical finally was banned.

In recent years the makers of cyclamate, Abbott Laboratories, and food and beverage trade organizations have been petitioning to put cyclamate back into our food supply.[8] (It is still used in about forty countries and can be bought in drugstores in Canada.) Studies continue to show, however, that in many people cyclamate breaks down into CHA, which is toxic to embryos and can atrophy the testicles as well as cause high blood pressure. So far, the American public remains protected by the FDA. A 1985 review issued by the National Academy of Sciences/National Research Council declared that the "suggestive" evidence must be fully investigated before the ban can be lifted.

ASPARTAME

Marketed as NutraSweet and the tabletop sweetener Equal, aspartame promised to be the answer to cyclamate—cheap, safe, and even sweeter on the tongue. The FDA approved the use of aspartame in 1981. Synthesized from two amino acids (aspartic acid and phenylalanine), this artificial sweetener is almost two hundred times sweeter than sugar. It contains as many calories as sugar, but only one two-hundredth as much is required to sweeten foods. Equal, however, uses sugar and dried corn syrup as a carrier to add bulk to the packet (and to make sugar addicts feel at home).

Aspartame is metabolized as protein, so it has no aftertaste— which may be the only good thing you can say about it. This time the FDA included a safety factor in its test procedures to determine "maximum allowable daily intake" rather than "average" intake. The amount decided on was no more than eight or nine aspartame-sweetened soft drinks for a child who weighs seventy-five pounds, and no more than seventeen such sodas for a 150-pound adult.

Soon after the introduction of aspartame, however, some users reported a number of bad reactions,[9] including rashes, headaches, and gastrointestinal upsets. G.D. Searle, aspartame's manufacturer, thought it had addressed any possible health hazard by pointing out on labels that phenylketonurics should not consume these products. Roughly one in 15,000 of us suffers from this metabolic disorder, in which the body lacks the enzyme needed to process one of aspartame's amino acids. In these people, phenylalanine can build up to toxic levels and cause, among other problems, brain damage. The condition is routinely diagnosed at birth, so Searle was acting to the good of at least a few Americans.

When aspartame decomposes, either in the can or bottle or inside your body, it releases methyl alcohol and a substance called DKP. While neither of these by-products has been implicated as a cause of aspartame-related illness, the fact remains that the sweetener's effects on the body have not been adequately tested. Two independent researchers, Richard Wurtman, a professor of biochemistry at MIT, and John Olney of Washington University in St. Louis, may have discovered why aspartame seems to cause mood changes and memory and sleep problems in many users. Their experiments indicated that aspartame interferes with neurotransmitters, chemicals that transmit messages between brain cells.[10] Therefore, the more aspartame you consume, the greater your risk of being out of sorts, being absentminded, and spending sleepless nights. The FDA dismissed Wurtman's and Olney's evidence as insignificant, however, and ignored Wurtman's claim it had acted in "unseemly haste" in approving the synthetic sweetener.

The FDA's opinion was subsequently supported by the American Medical Association, which claims aspartame is "safe for most people." Showing little more concern, the Centers for Disease Control, which analyzes consumer complaints about aspartame, declared it had not found "evidence for the existence of serious, widespread, adverse health consequences" to aspartame users. At this writing, in the face of mounting complaints, the CDC plans to schedule some long-delayed laboratory tests.

ACESULFAME-K

The most recent contender in the artificial sweetener sweep-stakes is acesulfame-K, marketed by an American subsidiary of West Germany's Hoechst A.G. With about the same sweetening power as aspartame, it claims as its advantages cheaper cost and greater stability. Called Sunette and, as a table sweetener, Sweet One, acesulfame-K is presently used in twenty countries, including France, Switzerland, the Soviet Union, and Australia.

But even before it came to the American marketplace in 1988, its safety was in question. In October of 1987, the Center for Science in the Public Interest sent the FDA results of two studies showing that animals fed acesulfame-K developed more tumors than animals not fed the chemicals. In another study provided by the CSPI, diabetic lab animals fed the substance showed abnormal rise in cholesterol blood levels.[11] The FDA, holding fast and planning no further tests, will no doubt change its collective mind if the complaints start coming in.

THE MYTH OF WEIGHT CONTROL

Even the FDA has to agree that artificial sweeteners are of no use in a reducing diet.[12] More than twenty years ago, animals fed cyclamates in amounts ingested by human beings put on pounds instead. What these sweeteners do is keep your sweet tooth alive and prevent you from learning to like less sweet, natural foods. And, speaking of teeth, the corrosive action of phosphoric acid in soft drinks, the most popular artificially sweetened product, can be as harmful to tooth enamel as sugar.

Synthetic sweeteners also delude us into thinking we're cutting down on calories, so why not have that piece of candy or cake? The more convincingly natural the taste, the more effectively they keep us hooked on the sweet and the fat. And, in the case of Equal and Sweet One, we're defeating our conscious purpose since both contain a gram of sugar in each serving. Artificially sweetened sodas have created a generation of sugarphobics who, like heroin users who switch to methadone, need their daily fix of a sweetener that is just as dangerous as the sugar they were hooked on. These were the people who objected hysterically when the FDA moved to ban saccharin in 1977. In reality, chemical analogues tend to create carbohydrate cravings that can be satisfied only with real sugar. It's a common sight to see one of these sugarphobics sip a can of diet soda while enjoying a dish of ice cream or a sugared doughnut.

The Evolution of Artificial Sweeteners

1879: A Johns Hopkins scientist hoping to find a wonder drug discovers saccharin instead. A noncaloric coal tar derivative 300 times sweeter than sugar, saccharin is soon found in a variety of canned foods.

1912: Tests indicate that saccharin is a carcinogen, prompting the fledgling Food and Drug Administration to ban its use as a food additive.

1914: To alleviate the sugar shortage of World War I, saccharin is declared safe for human consumption. Saccharin usage promptly increases as fast as the price of sugar, although it remains quietly suspect.

1937: Researchers working on a fever-reducing drug isolate from coal tar a sweet-tasting, nonnutritive chemical and call it cyclamate. Thirty times sweeter than sugar, cyclamate, unlike saccharin, produces no bitter aftertaste and can be used in cooking.

1950: The FDA approves cyclamate for food use. The following year, Kirsch Beverages introduces cyclamate-sweetened No-Cal and the diet soda industry is born.

1958: The Cumberland Packing Corp. introduces cyclamate-based Sweet 'n Low as a sugar substitute. Within five years, cyclamate, which is one-tenth the price of sugar, is used to sweeten canned goods, baked goods, toothpaste, mouthwash, cough medicine, bacon, cereal, and diet and nondiet beverages.

1965: While developing a new ulcer drug, a research chemist for G.D. Searle discovers aspartame, an amino acid compound 180 times as sweet as sugar.

1969: The FDA bans cyclamate when tests suggest that large doses cause bladder tumors in laboratory rats. Sweet 'n Low changes to a saccharin-based formula. Seven people bring a class action suit against the government for banning cyclamate.

1972: The FDA removes saccharin from its GRAS (Generally Recognized as Safe) list and puts limits on its use.

1977: When Canadian tests find that saccharin produces bladder tumors in laboratory rats, the FDA imposes a ban, to take effect in July. More than a million people write their representatives in support of saccharin, prompting Congress to impose a moratorium on the ban. Artificial sweeteners prove to be as addictive as sugar.

1981: Searle begins marketing aspartame as NutraSweet after the FDA approves its use in cold cereals, drink mixes, sugarless gums, gelatins, puddings, dairy products, nondairy toppings, and as a tabletop sweetener called Equal.

1983: The FDA approves aspartame for use in diet soft drinks. Congress extends its moratorium on the ban against saccharin to April 1985 (it is subsequently reextended).

1984: Although the American Medical Association concludes that saccharin and aspartame are safe for most people, the Massachusetts Institute of Technology identifies eighty-six people who suffered seizures after using aspartame. Tests indicate that saccharin may increase the risk of certain kinds of cancer in humans, and a warning label is put on products containing the sweetener.

1987: The FDA approves the use of aspartame in baked and cooked foods.

1988: West Germany's acesulfame-K arrives in the United States under the brand names Sunette and Sweet One. Consumer groups cite evidence that prolonged use of the sweetener can result in cancerous tumors, but the FDA declares it safe for human consumption.

1989: The search goes on for an innocuous artificial sweetener. Pfizer Inc. tests a new compound called Alutin which is ten times as sweet as aspartame; Johnson & Johnson tests another new synthetic sweetener. Others continue to investigate Miraculin, a low-calorie sweetener derived from a West African fruit.

15

Sweet Nothings

*"Tell me what you eat and I will tell you what your
are."*

—Anthelme Brillat-Savarin

THE ARISTOCRATS of Ancient Rome would have been very much at
home in contemporary America. With their taste for "essential
luxuries" and all-day Lucullan feasts, they would have eagerly
picked up the junk food habit, and added soft drinks, cookies,
cakes, and ice cream sundaes to their menu of sybaritic indul-
gences.

To judge from their rate of dental decay, the Romans may well
have been the original junk food addicts. From a starting point of
about 2,000 years B.C., the percentage of dental caries among
Romans was less than 3 percent. By the first century A.D., when
the Empire was near its peak, that rate had quadrupled to more than
11 percent.[1] A significant occurrence during those 2,000 years was
the invention of stone-milling, which made it possible for the
Romans to grind wheat into a creamy white powder from which
most of the grain's life-giving wheat germ and bran had been
removed.

Initially, white flour was eaten only by the wealthy, but as the
Empire became more affluent the poorer classes were able to afford
breads and sweets baked from this glutinous starch. Although
nutritionally unaware by our standards, the Romans knew from

practical experience that the whole grain was better for you. Gladiators and other athletes, for example, were fed bread made from the whole, dark meal because it made them healthier and stronger. Hippocrates, the father of medicine, sagely advised patients to eat bread made from unsifted meal "for its salutary effect upon the bowels."

Like many Americans, the Romans regarded eating as one of life's great sensual pleasures. Their taste ran to highly refined, highly flavored foods, which had the effect of overstimulating the appetite. Consequently, one helping of sweet-wine cakes from Africa, honey-soaked pastries from Greece, or rose-petal tarts fried in syrup was rarely enough to satisfy the patrician palate. The point of a Roman banquet of the late Empire was to savor and prolong the pleasure by eating as much of these rich dishes as you could hold. Dining for eight to twelve hours, however, can sorely test the physical capacity of the stomach. But the clever Romans solved this problem with a convenient remedy called the vomitorium. To keep the party going, all a diner needed to do was have a slave tickle his throat so he could regurgitate and begin eating all over again. The poet-philosopher Seneca described this cycle of goring and regorging as *vomunt ut edant, edunt ut vomant.* It was bulimia elevated to a high art.[2]

If the Romans had had our modern food surrogates they probably could have done away with the vomitorium. Technology has made it possible to create reduced-calorie and even no-calorie "foods" that mimic the real thing in taste, texture, and flavor. Synthetic flour, butter, sugar, colorings, and flavorings may not fool Mother Nature but they work remarkably well on the eyes and taste buds.

Why the Romans developed such a gluttonous taste for intensely flavored, sweetened foods as the Empire went into decline remains largely a mystery, although there are a few clues. One likely explanation, propounded recently in the scientific journals *Nature* and the *New England Journal of Medicine,* is that Rome was suffering from an epidemic of lead poisoning.[3] The lead had leached from lead pots commonly used in cooking and from the lead-based paint used to decorate pottery dishes and drinking mugs. Cato the Elder, a Roman statesman, records that vineyards also added "sugar of lead" (lead acetate) to sweeten their wines. Two of the symptoms of lead poisoning are loss of appetite and a metallic taste in the mouth. Perking up their palates and masking the taste of lead may well have been why the Romans ate as they did.

The ancient problem of lead poisoning has come back to haunt today. In 1988 we absorbed into our bodies more than one million tons of the deadly metal. Our air, food, and drinking water are all contaminated to varying degrees, compounding the risk of other industrial by-products floating insidiously through the environment. More than 17 percent of our children have levels of lead in their blood that exceed levels pediatricians regard as safe.[4] These children are at risk for long-term neurological damage, resulting in lowered IQs, school failure, dropping out, and antisocial behavior.

Lead, like refined sugar, does its dirty work slowly. The symptoms occur only after prolonged exposure and lead has accumulated in the tissues. A major source of lead poisoning among juveniles is house paint, which, prior to World War II, contained as much as 40 percent lead. Children living in older, substandard housing are at greatest risk, since at the age of two to about four they tend to explore their environments by tasting anything that comes their way. Chips of old paint peeling from walls and woodwork can look especially appealing.

But no American, rich or poor, escapes the risk of lead poisoning. Lead is also present in tap water, in canned foods, and in the air—from automobile exhaust, decaying car battery casings, and industries that use lead in their manufacturing process. An analysis of the dust in your house would probably reveal a high level of lead particles.

No single source of lead is likely to poison you by itself. But, like synthetic food additives, small amounts of lead absorbed from different sources can accumulate to toxic levels. When this happens, the capacity of hemoglobin, a substance in the blood that carries oxygen to the cells, is substantially reduced. Lead collects in the bone marrow, brain, and kidneys, further undermining their proper functioning. The symptoms of mild lead poisoning are surprisingly similar to those resulting from a diet high in refined carbohydrates (see Chapter 5): irritability, a decreased attention span, lethargy, stomach cramps, and constipation.

What part lead poisoning played in Rome's decline and fall— and in our own nutritional decline—has yet to be determined. While no single cause can explain such a complex event, it is worthy to note that Rome's earlier diet was quite different. For example, Rome's soldiers, the most powerful and well-organized fighting machine in the ancient world, subsisted largely on a diet of whole grain, cabbage, and whatever fruit and vegetables they could find. Meat and sugar, in the form of honey or date syrup, were eaten only occasionally. The Romans were so indebted to whole grains that they created a goddess of grain called Ceres. Her name survives in the word "cereal."

The foods we favor today, however, more closely resemble the diet of a later, decadent Rome. We are not about to give up our favorite, health-depleting foods any more than the Romans were. But what to do about the resultant plumpness, which in the ancient world was a mark of status and wealth? Our solution to the inherent contradictions of our national eating disorder is to conjure up mixtures of chemicals that can be eaten with pleasure while providing a minimum of nourishment.

The basic problem of devising a nonfood is that it either must have a molecular size large enough so that it isn't absorbed into the system, or, if it is absorbed into the bloodstream, it can pass out through the kidneys without having any effect on the body.[5] At this moment the food chemist has at his disposal all the ingredients necessary to fabricate any number of totally synthetic desserts that have little or no nutritive value. The recipe for a yellow cake, for instance, might include the following:

2 cups fluffy cellulose (for flour)
2 cups water
⅔ cup Olestra (for butter)
¼ cup saccharin (for sugar)
1 teaspoon vanillin (artificial vanilla)
⅛ teaspoon yellow dye
1 teaspoon baking powder

"Nonnutritive" isn't necessarily synonymous with bad, of course. The benefits of fiber, apple pectin, and alginate thickeners (made from seaweed) are well known. All are nondigestible substances that serve the purpose of cleansing the gastrointestinal tract, and some fibers help lower blood cholesterol. But the question is, what occurs in the system when a conglomeration of artificially created substances is taken into the body simultaneously? Moreover, since these chemicals were designed to substitute for our usual junk foods, they are likely to be consumed in excess.

Despite all evidence to the contrary, we cling to the notion that the food chemists will save us from our own excesses. The hard reality is that there is no safe alternative to the runaway consumption of sugar, fats, and white flour, nor is there ever likely to be one. Eating for pleasure at the expense of biological necessity may ultimately do us no more good than it did the Romans.

So far, the search for a perfect artificial sweetener has yet to yield a product that is any less harmful than sugar. Saccharin at one time seemed the perfect calorie-free sweetener because it is not modified by the body and passes unchanged into the urine. Saccharin is *absorbed* by the body, however, and was shown to cause cellular changes that can lead to cancer of the bladder. So we switched to cyclamate, which, although it tasted better, produced birth defects and kidney, liver, and bone marrow damage in other test animals. Now we have aspartame, which may cause brain damage, and acesulfame-K, which may cause tumors. Other new synthetic sweeteners are in the works.

The latest dieter's delight to come our way is fake fat. Procter & Gamble has led the race with its Olestra, a synthetic fat known generically as sucrose polyester (SPE), made by chemically binding ordinary table sugar to a string of fatty acids.[6] Sounding more like a wash-and-wear fabric than a diet food, this "no-fat fat" promises to revolutionize the American diet. Among its desirable properties, especially from a marketing point of view, is that it tastes and feels like the real thing. But unlike real fat, it has no artery-clogging cholesterol and passes through the body undigested.

Following on the heels of Olestra is NutraSweet's Simplesse, a cholesterol-free fat substitute derived from proteins in milk and egg whites.[7] Unlike Procter & Gamble's product, Simplesse is a reduced-calorie rather than a no-calorie "fat." Composed primarily of protein, it has 80 percent fewer calories than real fat and is digested and used like other nutrients.

Simplesse is actually one food disguised to look like another. NutraSweet chemists created the illusion of fat by extracting the protein from milk and egg whites, then heating, grinding, and blending the protein particles until they resembled the spheroidal shape of fat molecules. To the tongue, the resulting product feels as smooth and rich as real fat.

P&G's and NutraSweet's new goos are considerably different chemically and are slated for different uses by the food industry. If P&G's application to the Food and Drug Administration is any indication, the processed food giant plans to replace up to 75 percent of the fats used in fast food outlets and restaurants with Olestra, and to substitute it for up to 35 percent of the oils used in home cooking. Eventually, Olestra may turn up in everything from home-baked cookies to mayonnaise, French fries, and Oreo cookies.

The disadvantage of Simplesse is that it can't be used in frying or in most kinds of baking because it congeals the way egg whites do when heated. The drawback scarcely limits its many potential applications, however, and we will probably be eating it soon in such products as ice cream, salad dressings, yogurt, cheese spreads, and margarine. According to NutraSweet's spokesman, using Simplesse instead of fat in ice cream would bring an average serving down to 130 calories from 280, and salad dressings to 21 calories from 87.

Few things in life come without a cost, however, and fake fats are no exception. While Olestra has been shown to reduce the body's absorption of cholesterol, it may interfere with the absorption of vitamin A and other nutrients in the real food one would presumably eat with sucrose polyester. Some who have eaten the compound have experienced stomach cramps and diarrhea, and lab animals fed the substance have shown an increased incidence of liver problems, tumors, and leukemia.[8] A lower dosage might minimize these risks, but since it will be included in so many foods, it's not likely that millions of Americans will monitor their dosages.

Olestra is still undergoing a lengthy review by the FDA, a procedure that NutraSweet had attempted to sidestep by unilaterally declaring that Simplesse was by definition safe because it is "all natural." The FDA, beseiged by complaints from consumer groups, gave the public its customary nod and asked to see NutraSweet's test data.

The forward march of fake foods is no doubt inevitable, however, and it won't be long before Olestra and Simplesse work their way into America's diet. Before long, we will be able to combine these fats with a flour substitute called fluffy cellulose—compliments of the U.S. Department of Agriculture. Derived from sugar beet pulp and other agricultural waste, the ersatz flour may soon be replacing up to half the real thing in commercial breads and cakes.

Weight control is the principal reason most people turn to nonnutritive food and beverages, but the evidence is that nutrition-free products are ultimately self-defeating. Artificial sweeteners may produce an effect opposite to the intended one. The brain chemical serotonin, which is stimulated by sugar,[9] relays the message that enough sugar has been consumed. Artificial sweeteners neglect to carry this message, causing the brain to believe that more sugar or refined carbohydrates need to be eaten. With fake fat and fake flour added to fake sugar, it seems likely that many Americans will feel free to gorge themselves on their ersatz carbo-killers and continue to turn away from nutritious fruits, vegetables, and whole grains.

Those who suffer from advanced heart disease and high blood pressure, as well as the morbidly obese, might conceivably benefit from fat substitutes and by consuming fewer calories. Too much grease, sugar, and butter is probably the cause of their illness in the first place.

16

Candy in Your Medicine Chest

"There is a sucker born every minute."
—*P.T. Barnum*

NEXT TO THE supermarket, the drug store is America's busiest emporium. The two are usually situated close by and sometimes even within the same building. It seems a perfectly logical arrangement, given the fact that ill health induced by the former often leads one to the latter.

In 1987, Americans who "haven't got time for the pain"—in the words of one television commercial—spent $12 billion on over-the-counter nostrums and vitamin pills, or about 43 percent more than they did in 1982. There are now approximately 300,000 OTC products[1] on drug store shelves, packaged as pills, tablets, capsules, caplets, liquids, gum, and sprays. We can choose between "original" formulas, "new" formulas, and "advanced" formulas. For those who perceive they need it, there is an "extra-strength" product, or, if the condition is really severe, "maximum strength." Inspired by advertising claims and medical news, we all seem to be medicating ourselves to death in pursuit of an elusive goal of wellness.

While many OTC medications do work wonders in alleviating minor symptoms, none can correct the underlying cause of any illness. What our rush to the drug store indicates is a general decline in health and a blind faith in the ability of medical science to cure

151

all our ills. It's what the drug industry wants us to believe, of course. Profit not prevention is what has always been on the industry's mind—a situation not exactly conducive to the creation of a healthy, symptom-free America. Faulty nutrition, environmental pollution, urban stress, and lack of exercise have given drug manufacturers a captive market of millions. And the market will no doubt continue to grow.

Unfortunately, what we know about OTC medicines is what drug manufacturers choose to tell us. Advertising campaigns bombard us with gratuitous claims and paid testimonials about the efficacy of their products, which, it is claimed, will instantly remedy our particular malady. These sales pitches are often low-key and presented as educational messages, but their intent is to exploit rather than enlighten. Left out of the advertising hype is the fact that many of these magical elixirs are useless, unnecessary—and may even threaten your health.

How influential advertisements for OTC medications and health aids are was brought home several years ago by a study conducted by the FDA on American health habits. Among the questions presented to a representative survey group was: ''Do you agree that advertisements for over-the-counter medicines must be true or they wouldn't be allowed to say them?'' About 38 percent of the survey group responded yes.[2] When projected onto the population as a whole, that percentage translates into roughly fifty million Americans aged eighteen and over who believe the distorted claims of ceaselessly repeated, ubiquitous television commercials.

We don't need advertisements to tell us that Americans are beleaguered daily by various aches and pains, coughs, runny noses, upset stomachs, and sore throats. If left to its own devices, the body will heal itself, at least temporarily, but OTC drug manufacturers perceive, perhaps correctly, that we no longer trust our bodies to do the job. On television wives relieve their spouses' misery in seconds by administering the "pain reliever doctors recommend most." Cough syrups "go to work immediately" to provide a good night's sleep. Decongestants open stuffed-up nasal passages for all to see, thanks to the magic of animation. Antacid liquids and lozenges sweeten upset stomachs. And mouthwashes instantly banish germs that irritate mucous membranes.

It's no aberration that these products are among the industry's biggest sellers. All the symptoms they are designed to alleviate are the result of an immune system compromised by the unnatural stresses of everyday life. Why go to the trouble of removing the nutritional junk from your diet or trying to exercise more when you can pop a pill or a potion to mask the afteraffects of long neglect? But there is another, equally compelling reason consumers keep coming back to these products: they all contain copious amounts of sugar or other sweeteners.

The sparkly white crystals have spilled from supermarket shelves into a host of popular medications. Manufacturers routinely add sugar to their products for a number of reasons: as a preservative, a demulcent (to soothe irritated mucous membranes), and as an inexpensive solvent for colors and flavors.[3] In most cases, however, sugar is an unnecessary ingredient, added merely to add taste appeal to an otherwise bitter—and superfluous—medicine.

Although normally overlooked, hidden sugar in OTC medicines can add considerably to one's total daily intake, especially for the chronic patent medicine user. In the early 1970s, two research pharmacists at the State University of New York at Buffalo compared the glucose content of sugared medicines with people who took them and found that many were getting from 10 percent to 15 percent of their USRDA of carbohydrates from medications.[4] In other words, they were exacerbating their malaise by fanning the flames with yet more sugar. Their body's self-healing mechanism would have to overcome the effects of the sugar before going to work on the illness.

Even aspirin, that old reliable standby, seems more palatable to many when taken as a chewing gum called Aspergum. Advertised for "minor sore throat pain," Aspergum offers no topical relief for irritated membranes. Rather, it acts like every other aspirin does: it works when absorbed into the bloodstream from the small intestine. It tastes good, however, although at several times the price of common aspirin, it is cheaper to follow the advice of *Consumer Reports*: "Swallow an aspirin tablet—and then have a piece of sugarless gum."

Nearly as popular as aspirin are antacids, which are advertised as an antidote to a catchall malady called indigestion. Although the word has no medical meaning, it is commonly used to refer to many different irritations of the stomach. Gas, nausea, a bad cold, heartburn (the escape of stomach acid into the esophagus), emotional distress, and junk foods may all be at fault, but to a self-diagnostician, they all fall into the same category.[5]

Antacids work by coating the stomach with calcium carbonate and thus insulating it from the irritating factor. Treating oneself with antacids can be a risky proposition, for a stomach upset may indicate a more serious illness such as an ulcer or cancer, or may signal the imminent arrival of a heart attack. A sensible diet and reduction of stress would probably calm most troubled stomachs, but antacid tablets are quicker and as tasty as candy. The most popular brand, Rolaids, also happens to be the most heavily sweetened.

Even sweeter are cough drops and cough syrups. But here sugar has a proven pharmacological use. In a hard candy, which is essentially what a cough drop is, or a thick syrup, sugar clings to irritated throat membranes and gives them a chance to heal. If sugar weren't so addictive and we weren't consuming so much of it already, perhaps these products might be exonerated. But suppressing a cough may not be the wise thing to do anyway. Coughing is a reflex response to an irritation in the lungs or respiratory network. By defeating this protective response, you may be preventing the body from ridding itself of toxic secretions. Cough suppressants are particularly dangerous for those with lung diseases such as emphysema and bronchitis.[6]

Most OTC cough medicines are known in the trade as shotgun formulas, meaning they are compounds of three or four ingredients. The first is usually aspirin, the second a decongestant, the third an antihistamine. The fourth may be vitamin C or an antacid. Decongestants reduce swelling of the membranes of the nose and upper respiratory tract, and temporarily alleviate the stuffed-up feeling of a cold. But the membranes soon swell again, so the sufferer takes another dose. The result is rebound congestion, a swelling more severe than the original one. Drug makers, like the food adulterers down the block, want to keep you coming back for more. Stranger still are cough medications that contain an expectorant *and* a cough suppressant. Perhaps it makes sense to medicine makers to include a drug that makes phlegm easier to cough up in a product intended to make you stop coughing.

Since toothpastes and mouthwashes go into the mouth, manufacturers feel they have to sweeten these products too. The most common sweetener used is saccharin, which, although it does not cause tooth decay, may have even more dire consequences (see Chapter 14). Although these products are not swallowed, at least some residue makes its way into the stomach and is absorbed by the membranes of the mouth and throat. Another popular noncariogenic sugar substitute often added is sorbitol. Medically, sorbitol is used to increase the absorption of vitamins, but the dosage must be exact.[7] Too much and it hinders absorption and may cause diarrhea and gastrointestinal upsets. The FDA currently has sorbitol under review.

Probably the most useless personal hygiene product is mouthwash. Ever since Listerine coined the term *halitosis,* Americans have been falling for the line that bad breath has kept them from romantic and professional success. Listerine does kill a few germs (and is not sweetened), but most of these oral deodorants do nothing for bad breath except mask it with a flavoring oil. Among the ingredients you will find in a typical bottle of mouthwash are the following: sodium chloride, alcohol, water, sodium bicarbonate, zinc chloride, ammonium phosphate, propylene glycol, urea, boric acid, methyl salicylate, saccharin, and sorbitol.

The only beneficial ingredient in mouthwash is fluoride, a mineral made by dissolving tin in hydrofluoric acid. The chemical has been added to most municipal water supplies, and the result has been a rapid decline in tooth decay among children. According to the National Institute of Dental Research, part of the National Institutes of Health (NIH), nearly 50 percent of America's schoolchildren now show no evidence of tooth decay. Back in the early 1970s, that figure was only 28 percent.[8]

Fluoride, whether ingested from water, toothpaste, or mouthwash, is readily absorbed into the tooth enamel. It reconstitutes damaged surfaces and interferes with the conversion of sugar to acids in the mouth and inhibits the growth of harmful bacteria. It is a perfect antidote to the sweet, sticky junk foods that many children are reared on today. In this case at least, advances in medical technology have kept pace with our debased technological diet.

Hidden Sugar in Over-the-Counter Medicines[9]

Product	Percentage of Sugar
Benylin Cough Syrup	33.4
Cēpacol Throat Lozenges	50.6
Cheracol D	22.8
Chloraseptic cough drops	53.1
Coldene Adult Strength	28.7
Congespirin for Children	26.9
Coricidin	26.6
Creomulsion	3.7
Creo-terpin	5.4
Depree's Baby Cough Syrup	25.9
Dorcol Pediatric	11.1
Hall's Menthol-Lyptus Cherry	51.5
Hall's Menthol-Lyptus Honey Lemon	51.8
Hold—4-Hour Cough Suppressant	62.4
Listerine Cough Drops	68.9
Luden's Menthol Cough Drops	56.7
Luden's Wild Cherry Cough Drops	46.6
Pertussin—8-Hour	29.4
Pertussin—Wild Berry	28.3
Quelidrine	33.6
Recodene D	18.5
Riopan Antacid Chewable Tablets	12.7
Robitussin	3.3
Robitussin CF	0.7
Romilar—Children's	24.2
Sucrets—Cough Control	54.4
Sucrets—Sore Throat Lozenges	53.2
Sucrets—Sore Throat Lozenges for Children	58.9
Vicks Cough Silencers	22.0
Vicks Formula 44	20.1
Vicks Medicated Cough Drops	3.2
Vicks Medicating Throat Lozenges	66.2
Chewable Vitamins and Vitamin Drops	
Cheri-Dol Dolomite Tablets	39.2
Chewable Chocks	55.9
Chewable Vitamin E Tablets (Rugby Labs)	48.8
Deca-Vite Drops	3.4
Fluorac Multivitamins with Fluoride	7.8

Product	Percentage of Sugar
Poly-Vi-Flor Tablets	44.1
Poly-Vi-Sol Vitamin Tablets	21.0
Poly Vitamin Tablets	49.1
Vi-Daylin Tablets	26.3
Vi-Daylin with Fluoride Tablets	22.2

17

FDA Fudge

"No matter how tired and hungry and dry,
  The banquet how fine, don't' begin it
Till you think of the past and the future and sigh,
  'Oh, I wonder, I wonder, what's in it.' "
                                        —*Harvey W. Wiley*

DESPITE OUR post-Watergate and post-Vietnam skepticism, when the government speaks we listen, especially when the subject is our food supply. This is why food, beverage, and medicine manufacturers fight so hard to win the approval of the Food and Drug Administration. In theory, the FDA is supposed to be the vigilant guardian of the nation's health. But in practice the underbudgeted agency often allows manufacturers to make their own decisions as to what's good for the public. It's not surprising then that the sugar and artificial sweetener industries are the principal sponsors of studies concluding that these additives pose no significant threat to human health. A perusal of FDA case histories over the last two decades indicates that many similar findings are more than coincidentally related to the marketing needs of big business.

Sweetening up the nation's lawmakers keeps dozens of lobbyists for the sugar industry and its many clients gainfully employed in Washington, D.C. For several years, two of the capital's special-interest groups, the National Confectioners Association and the Chocolate Manufacturers Association, have been supplying sweets to the Senate at a desk in the back row of the Senate chamber.[1] The desk is conveniently located near the entrance through which most members come to vote and debate.

According to *The New York Times,* M & M Mars Inc., located in Hackettstown, New Jersey, routinely supplies the state's elected representatives with free candy. During the Reagan Administration, white boxes of M & Ms replaced gift boxes of cigarettes for guests aboard Air Force One, the President's plane. The boxes bore the President's seal, his signature in gold ink, and a cartoon version of an M & M candy holding an American flag. Similarly, Snack-PAC, the political lobbying arm of the Potato Chip/Snack Food Association, sends large gift tins of potato chips to selected members of Congress during the holiday season. Among those on SnackPAC's exclusive list are members of the House Education and Labor Committee, which decides what schoolchildren will be served in federal lunch programs.

Perhaps the snack food industry's most democratic giveaway is the annual Capitol Hill Ice Cream Social, described as the "biggest ice cream party in the world." Every June the International Ice Cream Association and the Milk Industry Foundation invites all members of Congress, and their staffs and families. In 1987 some 10,000 people attended the "social" to wolf down 2,500 gallons of ice cream, 5,000 cans of A&W root beer (for root beer floats), 250 gallons of Smucker's chocolate, butterscotch, hot fudge, and other toppings, and mountains of whipped cream and candy and coconut sprinkles.

Controlling the food and beverage business by means of legislation has always been easier said than done. The corporate world is a Goliath to the consumer's David, and it flexes considerably more muscle than the individual who eats its products. Among the consumer advocates currently aiming slingshots at the mighty giants is Dr. Sidney Wolfe, director of the Public Citizen Health

Research Group. Dr. Wolfe argues that the decisions of federal regulatory agencies are too often influenced by "pressures from the food industry trickling down through the White House, the Office of Management and Budget, the Secretary of Health and Human Services, and the Secretary of Agriculture. . . . Americans are not being adequately protected from cancer-causing or other dangerous substances in the food supply."[2]

The food industry generally regards Dr. Wolfe as a misguided annoyance, but it was just such a "crank" who goaded the administration and Congress into passing the first law prohibiting the adulteration of food and drugs. Back in the nineteenth century, wholesale and unpoliced tampering with food had become commonplace. The ripe yellow color of cheese often came from red lead; sulfate of copper kept pickles crisp and green; bitter almonds flavored dessert wines; and mineral dyes colored delectable cakes. Merchants routinely cheated consumers by watering milk, adding chicory to coffee, and barley to oatmeal. Bread was stretched with potato flour, chalk, whiting, or pipe clay; used tea leaves, bought from hotels and restaurants, were redried and colored with Prussian blue, black lead, and other poisons, and sold as new tea. Every year, these toxic additives took their toll in countless American lives.[3]

Rumors that some food processors were using ingredients that were poisonous had been circulating through the press for years. After several American soldiers died from eating poisoned canned beef during the Spanish-American War, newspapers and magazines began printing exposés of the food industry. Among those who zeroed in on the issue was Dr. Harvey W. Wiley, a dabbler in witty poetry and the chief chemist of the U.S. Department of Agriculture. Described as "the Ralph Nader of his day," Dr. Wiley decried impure foods in general, and was particularly outraged at the practice of "freshening" milk with such chemicals as formaldehyde and boric acid.

To prove that these preservatives were poisonous, Dr. Wiley assembled a group of "strong, robust fellows with maximum resistance to deleterious effects of adulterated food" and put them on a diet laced with chemicals. Each day his well-publicized "poison squad" ate foods with minute traces of commonly used preservatives and colorings. Sure enough, borax and boric acid, salicylic acid, sulfur dioxide, sulfate of copper, benzoic acid, and saltpeter sickened the men and caused many to lose their appetites. Dr. Wiley, aware of the expanding power of the media, issued regular bulletins to newspapers describing the ill effects caused by these additives.

With the help of popular publications that front-paged his poison squad experiments, Dr. Wiley managed to put together the nation's first consumer movement. At the same time, other writers were adding fuel to the fire by exposing the fraudulence and unsanitary practices of American food processors. The most significant among these was Upton Sinclair, whose galvanizing book *The Jungle* described in detail the filth surrounding the abattoir of most meat packers. In one chapter Sinclair described how meat handlers tossed scraps onto a blood-soaked floor, "then with shovels scraped up the balance" and mixed it into the good hamburger.

Although Dr. Wiley had little political clout, he did manage to convince a Nebraska senator to introduce a pure food law to Congress. The proposal was laughed down, however, prompting Dr. Wiley to take his case directly before the people. Witty and energetic, he organized his dedicated followers and sent them out into the field to collect signatures. With 10,000 petitions signed by their alarmed constituencies, Congress had no choice but to hold public hearings on the matter.

Finally, in 1906, President Theodore Roosevelt signed his approval to the Heyburn Act—America's first federal Pure Food and Drug Laws. Placed under the jurisdiction of the Agriculture Department, the laws were vastly watered down from the original regulations proposed by the bill's drafters. Many of Dr. Wiley's regulations were simply scratched out, which meant that foods sold to U.S. consumers still contained alarming ingredients with little or no restrictions. If he remained in the Agriculture Department, Dr. Wiley would be forced to abide by the new laws; rather than be muzzled, he resigned and once again took his case to the people. "Interest after interest, engaged in what the Bureau of Chemistry found to be the manufacture of misbranded or adulterated foods and drugs," he wrote, "made an appeal to escape appearing in court to defend their practices. Various methods were employed to secure this end, many of which were successful."[4]

In 1938 the Heyburn Act was expanded to the Federal Food, Drug and Cosmetic Act. In 1940 Dr. Wiley's Bureau of Chemistry was abolished and replaced by what is now called the Food and Drug Administration. (Contaminants and additives in meat and poultry remain the province of the Department of Agriculture.) While the 1938 law increased the authority of our watchdog agency, it was a 1958 amendment, the Delaney Clause, that has caused the most hand-wringing among food processors. Before the passage of this law, which took effect in March 1960, the FDA had no authority to remove from the marketplace any harmful additive unless it was contained in a product sold in interstate commerce.

The powerhouses behind the 1958 amendment were Representative James J. Delaney, a Democrat of Queens County, New York, and the legendary movie actress Gloria Swanson. After having his bill rejected by Congress five times, he enlisted the help of Swanson, who eagerly marched on Washington and convinced a group of Congressmen's wives to urge their husbands to vote for the amendment. Swanson, a living testimonial to the power of a natural diet, also convinced some of the wives to give up sugar, one of the "deadliest poisons" of all.[5]

Since the Delaney Amendment requires the food industry to prove that an additive does not cause cancer in humans or animals, it is not exactly to the food industry's liking. Critics claim that the Delaney cancer clause is too severe and that if were exposed to massive amounts of any substance we would probably all develop cancer. And since the clause doesn't cover other health problems like heart disease, high blood pressure, and liver and kidney ailments, why not strike it out altogether?

On the other hand, we have no idea of what the safe tolerances are for carcinogenic substances. Unlike the fast-acting poisons of Dr. Wiley's time, the sophisticated additives used today may work slowly and over a long period of time. No one dies after drinking one soft drink, but who knows what cumulative effect on health the soft drink habit will have over a lifetime. Therefore, why not err on the side of caution?

All such substances were removed from the agency's GRAS (Generally Recognized as Safe) list, and manufacturers were forbidden to use *any* amount of an additive shown to produce tumors in laboratory animals. The FDA's first compromise of the clause came in 1977, when it put a hold on its ban of saccharin. In 1981, a proposal to repeal the amendment by Senator Orrin G. Hatch, Republican of Idaho, fortunately died in committee. Finally, in 1985, after other abortive attempts to legislate the clause away, the FDA took it upon itself to reinterpret the clause—in favor of the food industry. Today the agency—which some in Washington call "Foot Draggers Always"—can allow cancer-causing agents in food if it determines the risk is minimal. Dr. Wolfe's Public Citizen group is currently fighting this unwarranted liberalization in court actions against the FDA.[6]

What is particularly disturbing about the FDA's waffling is that the agency seems to be turning a blind eye to the synergistic effect of the 3,000 or so chemicals routinely added to the manufacture of food and drugs.[7] Preservatives, emulsifiers, stabilizers, clarifiers, anticaking agents, antimicrobial agents, antioxidants, thickeners, colorings, and flavorings have all become part of our daily diet. What is needed is a radical new approach to testing that will take into account the interaction of substances in the total food environment, from pesticides in the ground to chemicals added by our food fabricators.

By trying to reassure the consumer while placating the food industry, the FDA has all but gotten lost in a morass of prolonged regulatory delays, litigation, and studies that have been planned but never made. As Dr. Donald Kennedy, the FDA commissioner during the Carter Administration, points out, "The budget has not grown to keep pace with the growth of responsibilities. But we have always tried to buy that particular service on the cheap."[8]

As could be expected, the history of the FDA is littered with incautious mistakes. Where was our trusted consumer surrogate when manufacturers decided to add sodium nitrate, monosodium glutamate, and sugar to baby foods? And why did it take so long to ban Red Dye No. 2, a coloring used in foods, drinks, and lipsticks, and said to cause cancer, spontaneous abortions, and birth defects? If not for independent studies and the action of vigilant consumer groups these chemicals probably would still be undermining the health of infants and their parents.

Still in our food supply is Red Dye No. 3, the replacement of Red Dye No. 2, which has been shown to cause thyroid cancers in laboratory rats. The artificial coloring can be found in soft drinks, ice cream, gelatins, baked goods, lipstick, rouge, salves, and face powder. Although the evidence against this chemical is strong, the FDA has put off making up its bureaucratic mind by planning a new study, which may take as long as three years. Among the study's sponsors are the cherry and pear industries, which are worried about the sales of fruit cocktail made from their produce. Red Dye No. 3 is the only food dye available that will color maraschino cherries without bleeding color into the other fruit. And many consumers, stated a spokesman for the California Pear Growers cooperative, will not buy fruit cocktail unless the cherries are dyed bright red.

Being on the GRAS list, of course, means that a chemical can be added to whatever food a manufacturer desires in whatever quantity it chooses. This is why salt and sugar, two of the most potentially dangerous additives of all, are sprinkled liberally in every food and drink imaginable. In 1986, after ten years of investigating the health effects of sugar, the FDA ultimately sided with the Sugar Association in absolving sugar from blame for a host of ills—except for tooth decay. The cookie monster, not to mention snack manufacturers, has apparently won after all.

At present the hired scientists of the food industry are still rigorously defending their chemicals on the grounds they are a socially acceptable risk. Not that they have much contest from the FDA and other regulatory agencies, whose unofficial slogan seems to be "see no evil."

Testing has been particularly lax in such recently introduced chemicals as aspartame, marketed as NutraSweet, which was approved for use in 1981 despite tests indicating that it produced brain lesions in mice. Instead of putting it on hold, the FDA overruled a board of inquiry and went on to allow the artificial sweetener to be used in more products. A petition by the Community Nutrition Institute, a Washington consumer group, to ban aspartame subsequently was rejected by a Circuit Court of Appeals. The FDA has grudgingly agreed to undertake more tests, but meanwhile Americans are consuming ever more of the questionable white powder.

Similarly, when Procter & Gamble introduced a fat substitute called Olestra, the FDA allowed the company to dispense with essential lifetime tests on laboratory animals. And when Monsanto's NutraSweet subsidiary came up with another fake fat called Simplesse and automatically put it on the GRAS list, the FDA responded with a mild rebuke that was little more than a slap on the wrist.

Sulfites provide yet another example of how the FDA's foot-dragging can result in tragedy. In 1982 the agency proposed adding sulfites to the GRAS list, in spite of studies uncovered by the Center for Science in the Public Interest which showed sulfites can cause asthmatic attacks. At the time sulfites were commonly used to keep the color in dried fruits and alcoholic beverages, and to prevent peeled raw potatoes and carrots from turning brown. It was not until six people had died from sulfite allergies that the FDA finally banned the chemical on most fresh fruits and vegetables. Sulfites in dried fruits and liquors must now be clearly labeled.[9]

Since most testing of additives is done by food manufacturers themselves, it is not inconceivable that hired researchers would have a vested interest in producing results their employers desire. The FDA is charged with the objective evaluation of this data and would seemingly take into account this built-in conflict of interest. But in practice, the agency too often gives in to the marketing needs of food and drug manufacturers and shirks the awesome responsibility resting on its shoulders. For now the American consumer will have to listen for the tiny voice of disinterested consumer advocates trying to make themselves heard over the din of advertising and public relations hype.

18

Shopping to Save Your Life

"If all the sugar were taken out of food, our super-markets would only need to be half as big."

—*Anonymous*

IF YOU WANT to understand the rights and wrongs of the American diet, you need only visit a local supermarket. There you will find the most varied, the cleanest, and the most readily available food supply in the history of the world. You will also find the sweetest, fattiest, most synthetic, and most nutritionally bankrupt foods man has ever had the misfortune to eat. And, you guessed it, these foods are a supermarket's biggest seller.

At least once a week we go there to spend our food dollars on items we and our families find appetizing. We rarely give much thought to nutritional value, and there is no one there to guide us through the aisles and tell us which foods we should be buying. Most of what we find on the shelves are products stocked from food processors interested only in profits. These products, with their jazzy packaging, promise unprecedented convenience, but this is more myth than reality. The major benefit of America's distribution system is not convenience but availability. Today, the year around, we can eat fresh vegetables grown in California, enjoy bananas grown in South America, have eggs without raising chickens, and buy oranges in the north, where they don't grow. We no

longer have to wait for the autumn harvest and then go to the trouble
of putting things by for the long winter.

If you are interested in squeezing the greatest nutritional benefit
from your food dollar (and you obviously are, if you have taken
the trouble to read this book), there are some things you need to
know about supermarket shopping. First, you should shop primarily along the perimeters of the store. The freshest and most
healthful foods are located along the walls. Here is where you'll
find fruit and vegetables, dairy products, chicken, fish and meat,
milk and other dairy products, frozen foods, and bakery counters,
many of which stock whole grain breads unpolluted by chemical
additives. Most supermarkets have a wide center aisle which is
designed to lure consumers there and to lead them past enticing
packages and cans of foods processed with tons of sugar and salt.
Another ploy is to purposely place dairy cases in a rear corner to
make certain you pass through the store.

Try to shop alone while the children are at school so that you
won't be pressured into buying junk food that your offspring have
seen advertised on television. Shopping by yourself also means
you will have enough time to compare prices, to analyze the
nutritional value of your purchases, and, above all, to read labels
and check their sugar content. Taking along a pocket calculator
will make the task easier and more efficient.

READING LABELS

Since 1938 food manufacturers have been obligated by law to
identify the ingredients for 350 common food products. Previously, consumers had no way of knowing that their canned goods
had been doctored with sugar, their coffee stretched with chicory,
and their fruit juice diluted with water. Today, manufacturers list

all ingredients in most processed foods in order of their weight, with the ingredients with the largest percentage listed first. In 1973, responding to consumer demand and threats by the FDA to have a new law passed, manufacturers voluntarily expanded labeling. The revised labels include the number of calories in an average portion of a product, the number of grams of protein, carbohydrates, and fat, and the percentage of vitamins and minerals, providing they are at least 2 percent of the U.S. Daily Recommended Allowance. The system requires no graduate degrees in statistical analysis to follow since it is based on the number 100.[1] You can even calculate the numbers in your head to determine how much nutrition you will be paying for at the checkout counter.

While this was a move in the right direction, and especially helpful to those counting calories, it is obvious that food manufacturers were still hedging. Labels still don't tell consumers everything they need to know and the information provided can be as misleading as it is confusing.[2] For example, few products tell whether the shortening inside them is saturated or unsaturated or whether these fats contain cholesterol. To find out, you have to read the fine-print list of ingredients and be aware of which oils are beneficial and which clog the arteries. Corn oil, olive oil, and soy oil are fine, but coconut and palm oils are more heavily saturated than butter and lard. Any products labeled simply "vegetable oils" should be avoided, since the oils referred to are probably coconut or palm, or a mixture of these tropical oils.

Additives pose another problem for label readers. While the majority of these must be listed among the other ingredients—making these products easy to avoid—coloring agents, spices, and flavorings do not. These may be described generically in this way: "artificial coloring," "artificially flavored," "with natural and artificial flavors," or, simply, "spices." Unless the manufacturer voluntarily reveals the sources of these substances, you have no way of knowing what they are derived from. For someone allergic to petrochemical-based additives or for those who react to natural colorings, flavorings, and spices, this presents a hidden health hazard.

For all its benefits, nutritional labeling tends to mislead the consumer into thinking processed foods are more nutritious than they actually are. Fresh foods and lightly processed foods, such as frozen fish and canned vegetables and fruit, provide a number of unlisted secondary vitamins and minerals, including folic acid, pyridoxine, vitamine B_{12}, zinc, copper, magnesium, and trace elements. In highly refined processed foods you are probably getting only what the list indicates and nothing more.

You will search in vain for labels that indicate what percentage of each ingredient the can or box contains. In other words, exactly how much chicken *is* in a chicken pot pie, and how much tuna *is* in a tuna noodle casserole? Manufacturers are loath to tell you and have consistently fought FDA attempts to legislate the inclusion of ingredient quantities on food labels.[3] Because of this lack of standardization when it comes to product labeling, the consumer is often the victim. While one side of the package lures you with imprecise claims that are not quite lies[4], the ingredient label, which may or may not provide adequate information, is all but hidden in small type on the back or bottom of the box. The claim ''low in fat'' or ''lower in fat'' has no restrictions, for example, unless applied to dairy products or meat. To check the actual fat content, you will have to scan the proportion list, then check the ingredient list to discover what kind of fat is used. Hoping to remedy this situation, Representative Jim Cooper, Democrat of Tennessee, has introduced a legislative package known as the Fair Food Labeling and Advertising Act. As you will see, this nutritional blackout can be particularly frustrating when trying to reduce or remove sugar from your diet.

SIFTING OUT SUGAR

Like a nutritional version of Gresham's law ("bad money drives out good"), the inclusion of sugar has become so widespread that it almost defies comprehension (see chart on pages 177–78). As far as food merchandisers are concerned, sugar and sweeteners are invaluable adjuncts to the manufacturing process. They can be used as preservatives, thickeners, to perk up inferior foods, to add bulk—and to addict the consumer. This makes sifting sugar from the diet difficult but not impossible, if you know how to read labels.

We all know that when sugar is at the top of the list it means there is more sugar in the package than any other ingredient. Therefore, some may reason, health risks are reduced if sugar is further down on the list, say in third or fourth place. What many of us are not aware of is the fact that manufacturers can use many different sweeteners in a single product. Whereas grains are often combined in a single listing, sweeteners are not, in order to keep refined sugar from appearing as the prime ingredient. For example, commercially prepared oat bran muffins and cookies (which suggest wholesomeness) may list sugar as the third ingredient, high fructose corn syrup as the fifth, and honey as the sixth. When totaled up, these sugars may well prove to be the primary ingredients.

A label stating that a product is "sugar free" is no guarantee that it is. Government regulations require only that such a product contain no refined sugar. Processed foods that contain fructose or glucose can be labeled "sugar free" even though they are as heavily sweetened and as high in calories as sucrose-sweetened varieties. The clever ways in which manufacturers can manipulate package labeling while remaining just this side of the truth can be seen in such products as Nabisco's 100% Bran. The box carefully points out that it contains "no artificial sweeteners" and that it is "flavored with two naturally sweet fruit juices." True enough. But there are also other sweeteners in the cereal and other ingredients besides wheat bran.

To reduce your intake of sweeteners—leading you, hopefully, to give them up—don't buy products that list sugar as one of their first three ingredients and which contain more than one kind of sweetener. Condiments like ketchup, mayonnaise, A-1 Sauce, Durkee's Famous Sauce, and sandwich spreads contain lesser amounts of sugar, and of course we use these in much smaller amounts. But if you want to improve your well-being, you had best seek out unsweetened varieties available at health-food stores—at least until you have kicked the habit.

Of all the hyped-up products that dominate supermarket shelves, the most nutritionally irrelevant are presweetened breakfast cereals and sweetened soft drinks. If manufacturers wanted to be totally honest, they would put warning labels on these items, which nutritionist Dr. Jean Mayer calls "semisynthetic" food. A skull and crossbones might be accompanied by the kind of caveat displayed on cigarette packages: "Danger! This product can be dangerous to your health" or "Eat and drink at your own risk." As with tobacco, a high tax could be imposed to defray the financial burden these products impose upon our health care system.

Cereal companies hammer away at consumers via television claiming their products are high in protein and fortified with eight essential vitamins and minerals. True enough. But which breakfast cereal isn't similarly fortified? And when did protein deprivation become a common problem in the United States? One brand claims it has no cholesterol, but which cereal does?

Many of these breakfast foods are more like candy than a cereal,[5] and children often pop them into their mouths throughout the day, without milk, as a junk food snack. Mom and Dad, having been inundated by magazine and newspaper articles, television news programs, and nutrition newsletters, probably know better, but they nevertheless continue to buy these breakfast cereals for their kids by the ton. Of course children like them, because they taste good.

Breakfast cereal was originally intended as a health food when Dr. James Caleb Jackson first concocted it about 125 years ago, to arrest "moral and physical" decline. Borrowing the coarse, whole grain flour promoted by the Reverend Sylvester Graham (inventor of the Graham Cracker), Dr. Jackson mixed graham flour with water, double-baked it, ground it up, and served it as a cold breakfast food mixed with fresh milk. He called it "granula." Later, Dr. John Harvey Kellogg, a vegetarian Adventist, promoted his corn flakes for health, and C.W. Post, a former Kellogg employee, was equally successful with a granula-like breakfast food called Grape-Nuts.

All these cereals contained the whole grain, and milling had not removed the bran (the fiber) or the niacin, thiamin, riboflavin, iron, and other nutrients contained in the germ, or seed. Today's breakfast cereals go through so many processing steps that these nutrients have to be put back in—and not all *can* be put back. Health-promoting grains such as corn, rice, wheat, and oats are now bleached, steamed, pressurized, toasted, flaked, puffed, artificially colored and flavored, coated with sugar, and preserved with chemicals. As for the vitamin enrichment, it is still true that, as consumerist Michael F. Jacobson noted nearly twenty years ago, "For their generosity in adding a half cent worth of vitamins to twelve ounces of cereal, they add 45 percent to the retail price."[6]

Adults eat lots of breakfast cereals too, so during the early 1980s cereal companies began pushing bran in addition to vitamin and mineral fortifiers. Overall, these adult cereals are more nutritionally sound than those pitched to children, but many contain more sugar than an adult would normally sprinkle on an unsweetened brand. Many up the ante by tossing in dried fruits such as raisins and dates. These have often been preserved with sulfites, which can cause breathing difficulties in those allergic to the chemical.

When buying breakfast cereals you can't go wrong if you stick to the old standbys sweetened with fruit, and, if you must, a tiny amount of sugar. Plain old Shredded Wheat is best, followed by Cheerios, Puffed Rice and Puffed Wheat, and Uncle Sam Cereal. Hot oatmeal packs a lot of food value and it is the least damaged by steel-cutting and rolling used in processing these cereal grains. Shredded Wheat and oatmeal have absolutely zero added sugar and preserve natural brans that can alleviate constipation and help prevent cancer of the colon. Oat bran has been shown to lower cholesterol levels. If you feed your child—or yourself—a fantasy product like Sugar Smacks, Cocoa Pebbles, or Lucky Charms, which are half sugar, you are not contributing to the health of people you love.

In the last ten years more than 10,000 new products have appeared on supermarket shelves, the majority of them convenience foods.[7] These products, according to a survey taken by researchers at Harvard University, are "distinguished by a remarkable lack of nutrients as the result of overprocessing. Overprocessing is the key. Add plenty of sugar and fat and you've got the . . . selling secret."[8]

SUPERMARKET SMARTS

The consumer movement has had some impact on the nation's supermarkets, although not enough to convince them to pressure food processors to eliminate added sugar from their products. But some chains, including Grand Union, Safeway, Giant Food, and Olson, point out what's in the package and how much of it is there.

Like Seattle's Olson chain, some 2,000 stores use Nutri-Guide, a shelf tag program based on guidelines from the American Heart and American Diabetes associations.[9] Others, like the Northeast's Grand Union chain, sport their own shelf cards that point out products low in sugar, sodium, and cholesterol and high in fiber.

All of these programs measure in grams, however, so in order to know just how much sugar you are getting, you will have to make the conversions yourself. Just remember that 4 grams of sugar equals one teaspoon; 12 grams equals one tablespoon. There are 4 calories in one gram of sugar. Therefore, if a product or product tag states that an average serving contains 24 grams of sugar, you are taking in 6 teaspoonsful, or 96 calories. Would you add that much yourself if you were composing the recipe? And remember, what's called an average serving is small, and that we usually eat more than the recommended portion.

These programs are a definite help when maneuvering through the supermarket minefield, but they still have a long way to go. It took ten years of consumer action by parents to get Virginia's Giant Foods to limit candy bars and chewing gum to only one lane per store.[10] So the sugar situation, it seems, is still desperate but not hopeless.

Sugar—From Soup to Nuts[11]
How much hidden sugar are we actually eating?

Product	Amount	Teaspoons of sugar
Doughnut, iced	1	6
Cupcake, iced	1	8
Brownie	1	3
Cream puff	1	5
Chocolate cake, iced	1/12 cake	15
Chocolate chip cookies	2 small	4
Chocolate bar	2 ounces	10
Fudge	1-inch square	3

Product	Amount	Teaspoons of sugar
Hard candy	2 ounces	8
Chewing gum	1 stick	½
Ice Cream	1 scoop	4
Sherbert	½ cup	6–7
Jello-O pudding	½ cup	4½
Kool-Aid	8 ounces	6
Soft drink	12 ounces	7–10
Tang	8 ounces	4
Orangeade	8 ounces	5
Chocolate milk	8 ounces	6
Milkshake	8 ounces	8–12
Hamburger bun	1	3
White bread	2 slices	1–2
Peanut butter	1 tablespoon	2
Jelly	1 tablespoon	3½
Peaches, canned, with syrup	2	3½
Apple sauce, sweetened	½ cup	5
Froot Loops	⅔ cup, dry	14
Kellogg's Raisin Bran	⅔ cup, dry	3½
Müeslix Five Grain	½ cup, dry	3
Instant Cream of Wheat, Brown Sugar and Cinnamon	½ cup, dry	3
Ketchup	1 tablespoon	1
Vegetable soup, canned	4 ounces	1½

19

How to Cure a Sweet Tooth

"Eating is self-punishment; punish the food instead. . . .
Throw darts at a cheesecake. . . . Beat up a cookie!"
—*Gilda Radner*

FIRST, the good news: kicking the sugar habit doesn't mean having to give up sweets. It merely means that you will have a new, truer conception of the word "sweet." Mother Nature has thoughtfully provided us with any number of tempting treats that contain no refined sugar, no white flour, and no artery-blocking fats. Once you have weaned yourself from processed treats, you are in store for a new taste sensation: the unadorned, untampered-with flavors of fresh and dried fruits, juicy ripe berries, fragrant nuts, and rich whole grain cereals. If you find you just can't give up cakes and cookies, you can make them yourself with the above ingredients and just a smidgen of sugar. You'll wonder what you ever saw in the store-bought variety.

Now, the bad news: You will have to give up an emotional crutch that has sustained you for years. You will have to say goodbye, perhaps forever, to soft drinks whether sugared or artificially sweetened, ice cream, corn chips, Twinkies, candy bars, and all the rest. Like an old but false friend, these junk foods have been undermining your good health for decades. Every time you chose a chocolate chip cookie over an apple or an orange or a slice of

179

whole wheat banana bread you were losing important vitamins, minerals, and fiber. You will find, as so many others have, that after your initial effort, the good points of kicking sugar vastly outweigh the pleasures of a bad habit. The sacrifice was all in your mind.

An effective way to start when you are kicking is to take a brisk ten- to fifteen-minute walk whenever your sweet tooth starts to ache. In an experiment by Dr. Robert E. Thayer, a psychologist at California State University at Long Beach, eighteen college students volunteered for a twelve-day study to find out which was more likely to relieve tension and restore energy: a candy bar or a rapid ten-minute walk. The students alternated between the two and rated their energy, tension, and tiredness levels after twenty minutes, one hour, and two hours.

Overall, the students discovered they felt much more energetic and less tired after the walk than after munching on the snack. The effect held true for all time periods. On days they ate the candy, most students experienced a quick energy pickup that all but vanished after two hours. Their tension subsequently began to increase. "It may be commonly known that sugar causes a pickup followed by a decline in energy," Thayer concluded. "What is not known by most people is that even a very small amount of exercise can be energizing. And this type of energy is relatively free of the tension brought on by sugar."[1]

BEVERAGES

Forget about diet sodas, which are as nutritionally bankrupt and as harmful as sugared soft drinks. Water is still our best thirst-quenching beverage, and it has no calories. To make your water more appetizing, keep it ice cold in the refrigerator in an attractive container. Unsalted club soda is the next best choice, and you can flavor it with a slice of lemon or orange, or make an apple or orange soda by adding a jigger of apple or orange juice. In no time at all, you will find that most soft drinks taste nauseatingly sweet.

FRUIT

Fresh fruit not only tastes good, it may help cut the risk of stroke nearly in half by increasing the body's supply of potassium. This is the conclusion of a study conducted by Dr. Elizabeth Barrett-Connor of the University of California at San Diego. Dr. Barrett-Connor connects the declining stroke rate in the United States with the increased availability of fresh fruit since the late 1940s. ''The results indicate that one extra serving of fresh fruits or vegetables each day may decrease the risk of stroke by as much as 40 percent, regardless of other factors,'' Dr. Barrett-Connor said.[2] Since stroke remains the nation's third leading cause of death—after heart disease and cancer—this is indeed good news. In 1988 more than 150,000 people died of a stroke.

Bananas are particularly rich in potassium, and they can be eaten a number of ways: plain, sliced into a bowl of milk or cereal, or frozen into a close approximation of a popsicle.

Grapefruit has also been shown to have unsuspected benefits in lowering cholesterol levels that lead to arterial disease. Researchers at the University of Florida at Gainesville reported that grapefruit pectin, the substance that binds cell walls, also binds with bile acids to reduce cholesterol in the blood.[3] These pectins are especially prevalent in the rinds and fleshy parts of citrus fruits. Pectin, of course, is what grandma used to make her jelly jell.

While apples may not keep the doctor away, they will probably help reduce your medical bills. Apples also have the type of fiber called pectin, which lowers cholesterol.[4] The fiber and bulk and natural sweetness of an apple can satisfy the most demanding sweet tooth. You can even use an apple as a sweetener by grating it over your cereal in the morning. An experiment at the University of Bristol in England has shown that the pectin in apples helps prevent overeating by drawing only moderately on your insulin bank. Blood sugar levels return to normal fairly quickly after eating an apple, and you are not left with the hunger pangs associated with rebound hypoglycemia.

But remember to buy apples which have not been treated with daminozide, a chemical marketed under the trade name Alar. A growth regulator used to make apples ripen uniformly and stay crisp in storage, Alar and the toxic by-product it produces when treated apples are eaten may increase your risk of cancer.[5] The Environmental Protection Agency has ordered it off the market by 1991, but until then about 15 percent of the U.S. apple crop is being treated with the chemical. Washing will remove most of the wax fruit growers unfortunately coat their products with, but nothing can remove the Alar from treated apples.

Raspberries, strawberries, and blueberries are the royalty of the fruit world and as such don't really require an adornment. But if your soul cries out for heavy cream, try circumventing your taste buds with a little imagination. Equal parts of cottage cheese and plain yogurt whipped in a blender will produce a rich, creamy substitute.

The next best alternative to fresh fruit is sun-dried fruit. Sun-drying has been a common practice since ancient times, when fruits and vegetables were put by in cold and temperate zones for the coming winter. Fresh fruits contain many vitamins, minerals, and enzymes as well as the readily absorbable simple sugars, fructose and glucose. During the drying process, some of these nutrients are altered and the sugar content increases. The most commonly available dried fruits are apricots, grapes (raisins), plums (prunes), dates, figs, and apples. Commercially produced dried fruits are usually not sun-dried but dehydrated by chemicals and treated with sulfites to preserve their color. In some people, sulfites can produce dangerous allergic reactions.

Speaking of prunes, these much maligned wrinkled plums are among the richest sources of dietary fiber. About two ounces of dry pitted prunes yield approximately nine grams of fiber. Furthermore, prunes contain several types of fiber, including cellulose, hemicellulose, lignin, and pectin. They are also especially high in potassium and vitamin A and contain calcium. As with dates and dried figs, you can eat prunes whole, add them to cereal, or chop them up to bake in whole grain muffins.[6]

NUTS AND SEEDS

Botanically, a nut is a one-seeded fruit, as in the chestnut, acorn, and hazelnut. Most of what we call nuts are actually something else. The pecan and walnut are fruits, the cashew, Brazil nut, and pistachio are seeds, and the peanut is a bean. In many parts of the tropical and subtropical world, nuts are a staple food. And what keeps African and South American natives healthy will probably do the same for you. Nuts are packed with nutrition and contain about twice the amount of nutrients supplied by any other foodstuffs their size.[7] They are a good source of protein and contain copious amounts of unsaturated oils.

All nuts contain vitamin E, some of the B complex group, and assorted minerals. Nutritionists recommend them as a choice substitute for sweet and starchy snacks, since they also benefit the cardiovascular system. Unsweetened peanut butter on a whole wheat cracker is immensely satisfying. But all nuts are high in calories, so if you eat too many of these tiny powerhouses you will almost certainly gain weight.

Pumpkin and sunflower seeds are widely available in health food stores, where you may find other naturally tasty snacks. (But be careful: many so-called health food products are as heavily sugared as supermarket varieties.) The seeds are a staple in the Middle East, where they are eaten whole or ground into a flour and used in baking. They are both high in essential nutrients, and can be popped into the mouth like potato and corn chips.

WHOLE GRAINS

Processed food manufacturers haven't quite transformed every cereal into candy-coated puffs. The have left their meddling hands off oatmeal, Shredded Wheat, farina, and Cream of Wheat, among others. Skim or part-skim milk will add to the natural sweetness of these grains, but if you crave something stronger, sliced fruit will do the trick.

All of the above-mentioned ingredients can be combined into a nutritious whole dessert like the following, which never fails to please a recovering sugarholic:

Walnut Treats

2	egg whites
9	dates
½	cup walnut halves
5	heaping tablespoons whole wheat flour
1	tablespoon wheat germ
½	cup unsulfured raisins
½	cup unsulfured sultanas
2	teaspoons fructose
½	teaspoon powdered cinnamon
¼	teaspoon ground nutmeg

Beat the egg whites until they hold a soft point when the beater is raised. Chop dates coarsely and mix together all ingredients. Form into 16 balls. Place on a greased cookie sheet and bake for 15 minutes in a 350° Fahrenheit oven. Remove from oven and allow to cool. Wrap each treat in plastic wrap.

This recipe is adapted from Yvonne Young Tarr's *The New York Times Natural Foods Dieting Book,* which offers a wide range of recipes for healthful, eminently satisfying desserts. Another good source of recipes is Ellen Buchman Ewald's *Recipes for a Small Planet.*

LAST WORDS

- Never bring candy or junk snack foods into the house "to have when guests visit." You are lying to your best friend—yourself. Sooner or later, like an alcoholic who has a bottle stashed in the closet, you will succumb.
- Don't think of sweets as a reward for yourself or your children. Instead, try to think of sugary food as an addictive drug that has been punishing your body for many years.
- Read labels carefully when shopping for food to make certain you are not getting any added sugar. Remember, it's the cumulative effect that hurts.
- Perk up foods with sweet spices and herbs, such as cinnamon, ginger, coriander, and nutmeg. A sprinkling of chopped nuts or coconut will also add natural sweetness.
- Gradually reduce the amount of sugar you use in your coffee or tea until you are using none at all.
- Remember that quitting isn't an act, it's a process. Getting sugar out of your system does not require an enormous effort

of will. Quitting requires only organized motivation. The knowledge you have derived from this book will give you power to free yourself—forever—from your rotting sweet tooth.

- Don't be put off if your resolve crumbles when you are beginning to kick the habit. An Oreo cookie or chocolate ice cream binge isn't the end of the world. Don't dwell on feelings of inadequacy such as "I guess I just don't have the will power." Instead, resolve to stay away from temptation and develop a positive addiction to take the place of sugar. Reward yourself with time spent at a pleasurable activity such as jogging, walking, tennis, or gardening.

- Keep in mind that you will be reducing your risk of premature death from heart disease, stroke, and other leading causes of death, while ameliorating the vigor-depriving syndromes associated with excess sugar consumption.

- Look in the mirror and congratulate yourself on the pounds you have lost. You will feel and look better than you have in years.

Notes

1. *Eat Now, Die Later*

1. *The Surgeon General's Report on Nutrition and Health*, Washington, D.C., June, 1988; The American Heart Association.

2. Stated by Martha Pehl, R.N., a representative of the Sugar Association, on the television program *Contemporary Health Issues*, aired by the Public Broadcasting System on February 13, 1983.

3. *The Evaluation of Health Aspects of Sugars Contained in Carbohydrate Sweeteners*. Report of the Sugar Task Force (Washington, D.C.: FDA, 1986).

4. U.S. Department of Agriculture, Economic Research Service.

5. Joseph Carey, "A Study of Sugar Stirs Up a Sweet-and-Sour Reaction," *U.S. News & World Report* 19 Jan. 1987.

6. Ross Hume Hall, *Food for Nought: The Decline in Nutrition* (New York: Harper & Row, 1974).

7. Richard Borshay Lee, *¡The Kung San.* (Cambridge, England: Cambridge UP, 1979).

8. Leonard A. Cohen, "Diet and Cancer," *Scientific American* November 1987.

9. Boyd Eaton and Melvin J. Konner, "Paleolithic Nutrition: A Consideration of Its Nature and Current Implications," *New England Journal of Medicine* 31 Jan. 1985.

2. *The Fat of the Land*

1. Warren E. Leary, "Young Women Are Getting Fatter, Study Finds," *New York Times* 23 Feb. 1989.

2. Leary.

3. "New Weight Standards for Men and Women," *Statistical Bulletin of the Metropolitan Life Insurance Company* (1980).

4. U.S. Department of Health, Education and Welfare, ''Weight by Height and Age for Adults 18–74 Years, United States, 1971–1974,'' *Vital and Health Statistics* (1979).

5. Richard E. Keesey, ''A Set-Point Analysis of the Regulation of Body Weight,'' in *Obesity*, ed. Albert Strunk (Philadelphia: Saunders, 1980).

6. P. C. Boyle, L. H. Storlien, and R. E. Keesey, ''Increased Efficiency of Food Utilization Following Weight Loss,'' *Physiology and Behavior* 21 (1978).

7. ''Gallbladder Risk Tied to Ice Age Ancestors,'' *New York Times* 19 June 1988.

8. Diana Tonnessen, ''Sugar Stand-ins,'' *Health* December 1988.

9. David R. Jacobs, Jr., and Sara Gottenborg, ''Smokers Eat More, Weigh Less than Nonsmokers,'' *American Journal of Public Health* 71 (1981).

10. Covert Bailey, *Fit or Fat?* (Boston: Houghton Mifflin, 1977).

3. *The Candy-Coated Teat*

1. U.S. Department of Health and Human Services, *Health, United States, 1986.*

2. *American Journal of Public Health* 78 (1988).

3. Bonnie Liebman, ''The All-American Junk Food Diet,'' *Nutrition Action Healthletter* May 1988.

4. Liebman.

5. *Journal of Broadcasting & Electronic Media* 32 (1988).

6. Action for Children's Television (ACT), Washington, D.C.

7. U.S. Department of Agriculture, *National Food Situation* (1986).

8. National Center for Health Education, New York City.

4. *Sugar: An Unnatural History*

1. L.A.G. Strong, *The Story of Sugar* (London: George Weidenfeld & Nicolson, 1954).

2. G. N. Bollenback, "The Sweet Story of Sugar's Amazing Healing Powers," *Nutrition Today* January–February 1986.

3. Reay Tannahill, *Food in History* (New York: Stein & Day, 1973).

4. Noel Deerr, *The History of Sugar* (London: Chapman & Hall, 1949).

5. James Gorman, "Sweet Toothlessness," *Discover* October 1980.

6. Daniel J. Boorstin, *The Americans: The Democratic Experience* (New York: Random House, 1973).

7. Strong, *Story.*

8. Clyde H. Farnsworth, "Buried in '87 Spending Law: Easing of Sugar Imports Cuts," *New York Times* 6 Jan. 1988.

5. *Me, a Sugarholic?*

1. Carlton Fredericks, *Nutrition Guide for the Prevention and Cure of Common Ailments and Diseases* (New York: Simon & Schuster, 1982).

2. Roland Barthes, "Toward a Psychosociology of Contemporary Food Consumption," in *Food and Drink in History* (Baltimore: Johns Hopkins UP 1979).

3. Eccleston, D., "The Biochemistry of Human Moods," *New Scientist* 4 Jan. 1973.

4. Harold M. Schmeck, Jr., "Depression and Anxiety Seen As Cause of Much Addiction," *New York Times* 15 Nov. 1988.

5. National Institute of Mental Health (NIMH), 1987.

6. National Institute.

7. General Services Administration, *National Health and Nutrition Examination Survey (HANES): 1976–80* (1988).

8. Hilde Bruch, *Eating Disorders* (New York: Basic Books, 1973).

9. William Bennett, M.D., and Joel Gurin, *The Dieter's Dilemma* (New York: Basic Books, 1982).

6. *Sugar Stress*

1. E. M. Abrahamson, *Body, Mind and Sugar* (New York: Pyramid Books, 1971).

2. Abrahamson.

3. Richard A. Passwater, *Supernutrition* (New York: Pocket Books, 1976).

4. Adrenal Metabolic Research Society, *Hypoglycemia and Me?* (Mount Vernon, NY, 1970).

5. Roger J. Williams and Dwight K. Kalita, eds., *A Physician's Handbook on Orthomolecular Medicine* (New York: Pergamon Press, 1977).

6. Carlton Fredericks and Herbert Bailey, *Food Facts & Fallacies* (New York: Arc Books, 1971).

7. E. Cheraskin and W. M. Ringsdorf, Jr., *Psychodietetics* (Briarcliff Manor: Stein & Day, 1974).

7. *Grazing in the Wrong Pastures*

1. U.S. Department of Agriculture, Economic Research Service, *Historical Statistics, Colonial Times to 1989.*

2. U.S. Department of Agriculture, Economic Research Service.

3. Joseph Pereira, "The Exercise Boom Loses Its Strength," *Wall Street Journal* 9 Jan. 1989.

4. Trish Hall, "Self-Denial Fades As Americans Return to the Sweet Life," *New York Times* 11 Mar. 1987.

5. Andy Warhol, "Secrets of My Life," *New York* 31 Mar. 1975.

6. Eric Asimov, "The Heath Bar Finds Its Métier: Ice Cream," *New York Times* 19 Aug. 1987.

7. Corby Kummer, "America Is Going Sweet on White Chocolate," *New York Times* 21 Dec. 1988.

8. National Confectioners Association, press release (1987).

9. Trish Hall, "Now, Food for the Otherwise Engaged," *New York Times* 15 Apr. 1987.

10. Marian Burros, "What Americans Really Eat: Nutrition Can Wait," *New York Times* 6 Jan. 1988.

8. *The Fast-Food Lane*

1. U.S. Bureau of the Census, *U.S. Census of Business* and *Survey of Current Business.*

2. John F. Mariani, *The Dictionary of American Food and Drink* (New York: Ticknor & Fields, 1983).

3. Max Boas and Steve Chain, *Big Mac: The Unauthorized Story of McDonalds* (New York: Dutton, 1976).

4. "How Nutritious Are Fast Food Meals?" *Consumer Reports* May 1975.

5. Extrapolated from figures published by the U.S. Department of Agriculture's *National Food Situation*; National Candy Wholesalers Association; National Soft Drink Association; and the Roper Organization.

6. "The Lure of Fast Foods," *American Journal of Psychiatry* August 1979.

7. *Wholesome Diet* (New York: Time-Life Books, 1981).

8. H. A. Schroeder, *Trace Elements and Man* (Old Greenwich: Devin-Adair, 1974).

9. "Roy Rogers, Out to Lunch," *New York Times*, 19 Sept. 1988.

9. *The Osteoporosis Explosion*

1. National Institute of Arthritis and Musculoskeletal and Skin Diseases (1987).

2. National Osteoporosis Foundation (1987).

3. National Soft Drink Association (1987).

4. "A Morning Cola Instead of Coffee?" *New York Times*, 20 Jan. 1988.

5. Jane E. Brody, "Personal Health," *New York Times* 13 May 1987.

6. National Soft Drink Association (1987).

7. Brody, "Personal."

8. H. Spencer, "Osteoporosis: Goals of Therapy," *Hospital Practice* March 1982.

10. *A Feast for Yeast*

1. *The Physicians' Manual for Patients* (New York: Times Books, 1984).

2. C. O. Truss, "Metabolic Abnormalities in Patients with Chronic Candidiasis—The Acetaldehyde Hypothesis," *Journal of Orthomolecular Psychiatry,* 13.2 (1984).

3. C. O. Truss, *The Missing Diagnosis* (Birmingham, 1983). Privately published.

4. Truss, *Missing.*

5. William G. Crook, M.D., *The Yeast Connection* (New York, Vintage Books, 1986).

6. Ross Trattler, *Better Health Through Natural Healing* (New York: McGraw-Hill, 1985).

7. Jane E. Brody, "Personal Health," *New York Times* 8 April 1987.

11. *The Major Killers*

1. *International Lists of Diseases and Causes of Death,* U.S. National Center for Health Statistics; United Nations Statistical Office, New York.

2. Hall, *Food.*

3. American Diabetes Association, New York.

4. B. E. Lowenstein, *Diabetes* (New York: Harper & Row, 1976).

5. Frederick G. Banting, *Strength and Health* May–June 1972.

6. Jane E. Brody, "Dietary Fat Linked to Breast Cancer," *New York Times* 7 Mar. 1989.

7. American Cancer Society (1987).

8. Richard Borshay Lee, *¡The Kung San* (Cambridge, England: Cambridge UP, 1979).

9. Reuel A. Stallones, "The Rise and Fall of Ischemic Heart Disease," *Scientific American* May 1980.

10. U.S. Department of Agriculture, Economic Research Service, *Historical Statistics, Colonial Times to 1980.*

11. John Yudkin, M.D., *Sweet and Dangerous* (New York: Wyden, 1972).

12. Anthony Sclafani and Deleri Springer, ''Dietary Obesity in Adult Rats,'' *Physiology and Behavior* 17 (1976).

12. *Natural Foods or Nutritional Traps?*

1. Karen Croke, ''Telling It Like It Isn't Quite,'' *New York Daily News* 1 Feb. 1989.

2. U.S. Department of Agriculture, Economic Research Service (1987).

3. ''Buying Guide: Yogurt,'' *University of California, Berkeley Wellness Letter* June 1987.

4. Rafael Macia, *The Natural Foods and Nutrition Handbook* (New York: Perennial Library, 1972).

5. Marian Burrow, ''Oat Bran: The Muffin and the Mania,'' *New York Times* 26 Oct. 1988.

6. ''Salad Bar Smorgasbords,'' *Nutrition Action Healthletter,* March 1988.

7. John F. Mariani, *The Dictionary of American Food and Drink* (New York: Ticknor & Fields, 1983).

8. Macia, *Natural.*

9. ''Frozen Desserts: What's the Scoop?'' *University of California, Berkeley Wellness Letter* June 1989.

13. *Addiction Times Two*

1. ''Coming to Grips with Alcoholism,'' *U.S. News & World Report* 30 Nov. 1987.

2. National Institute on Alcohol Abuse and Alcoholism (1986).

3. R. J. Williams, *Nutrition Against Disease* (New York: Pitman, 1971).

4. U. D. Register, et al., "Influence of Nutrients on the Intake of Alcohol," *Journal of the American Dietetic Association* August 1972.

5. *Medical World News* 16 Mar. 1973.

6. Bill Keller, "Soviet Rations Sugar in Move to Foil Moonshiners," *The New York Times,* 27 Apr. 1988.

7. Anne Montgomery, "The Cooler Illusion," *Nutrition Action Healthletter* August 1988.

8. Alison Leigh Cowan, "A Weaker Market for Coolers," *New York Times,* October 19, 1987.

9. L. D. Johnston, et al., *Drug Use Among American High School Students, College Students, and Other Young Adults: National Trends Through 1985* (Rockville: National Institute on Drug Abuse, 1986).

10. National Cancer Institute, "Alcohol Consumption and Breast Cancer in the Epidemiology Follow-up Study," *New England Journal of Medicine,* May 7, 1987.

11. "Coming to Grips."

14. *The Truth About Artificial Sweeteners*

1. James Trager, *The Food Book* (New York: Grossman, 1970).

2. O. E. Anderson, *The Health of a Nation: Harvey W. Wiley and the Fight for Pure Food* (Chicago: Chicago UP, 1958).

3. *Wholesome Diet* (New York: Time-Life Books, 1981).

4. *The New Medicine Show* (Mount Vernon: Consumer Reports Books, 1989).

5. Michael F. Jacobson, *Eater's Digest* (Garden City: Doubleday, 1972).

6. Magnus Pike, *Synthetic Food* (London: John Murray 1972).

7. Jacobson, *Eater's.*

8. "Sweetener Ban May Be Overturned," *Insight* 19 June 1989.

9. "How Safe Is Aspartame?" *University of California, Berkeley Wellness Letter* February 1987.

10. *The New Medicine Show.*

11. "New Artificial Sweetener Not So Sweet," *Nutrition Action Healthletter* September 1988.

12. FDA, *How to Take Weight Off Without Getting Ripped Off* (Washington, D.C.: 1985).

15. *Sweet Nothings*

1. G. Daniel, ed., *Bones, Bodies and Disease* vol. 37, *Ancient People and Places* (London: Thames and Hudson, 1964).

2. James Trager, *The Food Book* (New York: Grossman, 1970).

3. Richard Wedeen, *Poison in the Pot: The Legacy of Lead* (Carbondale: Southern Illinois UP, 1984).

4. Environmental Defense Fund, Washington, D.C. (1988).

5. Magnus Pike, *Synthetic Food* (London: John Murray, 1972).

6. Calvin Sims, "Nutrasweet Reports Fat Substitute," *New York Times* 28 Jan. 1988.

7. Sims, "NutraSweet."

8. Elaine Blume, "Finessing Fat," *Nutrition Action Healthletter* November, 1987.

9. J. J. Wurtman, "Ways That Foods Can Affect the Brain," *Nutrition Reviews* May 1986.

16. *Candy in Your Medicine Chest*

1. Food and Drug Administration (1988).

2. *The New Medicine Show* (Mount Vernon: Consumer Reports Books, 1989).

3. Ruth Winter, *A Consumer's Dictionary of Food Additives* (New York: Crown, 1972).

4. E. Cheraskin and W. M. Ringsdorf, Jr., *Psychodietetics* (Briarcliff Manor: Stein and Day, 1974).

5. Carlton Fredericks, *Nutrition Guide for the Prevention and Care of Common Ailments and Diseases* (New York: Simon & Schuster, 1982).

6. *The New Medicine Show*.

7. Ruth Winter, *Consumer's*.

8. "Survey Finds Sharp Drop in Tooth Decay for Children in U.S." *New York Times* 22 June 1988.

9. Sources: American Dietetic Association; *Consumer Reports;* Food and Drug Administration.

17. *FDA Fudge*

1. "Sweetening the Senate," *New York Times* 25 Apr. 1988.

2. Marian Burros, "U.S. Food Regulation: Tales From a Twilight Zone," *New York Times* 10 June 1987.

3. O. E. Anderson, *The Health of a Nation: Harvey W. Wiley and the Fight for Pure Food* (Chicago: Chicago UP, 1958).

4. Harvey W. Wiley, *The History of a Crime Against the Food Law*, published by the author (Washington, D.C., 1929).

5. James Trager, *The Food Book* (New York: Grossman, 1970).

6. Marian Burros, "Oat Bran: The Muffin and the Mania," *New York Times* 26 Oct. 1988.

7. The Center for Science in the Public Interest, Washington, D.C. (1988).

8. Marian Burros, "Oat Bran."

9. Environmental Protection Agency, press release (1986).

18. *Shopping to Save Your Life*

1. FDA, *Consumer's Guide to Food Labels* (1983).

2. Stephen B. Schmidt, "Reform Food Labels Now!" *Nutrition Action Healthletter* March 1989.

3. "Telling What's in Your Food," Reuters news service, May 31, 1988.

4. "FDA Faulted for Shift on Food Label Rules," *New York Times* 13 Apr. 1988.

5. Center for Science in the Public Interest *Sugar Scoreboard,* (Washington, D.C., 1983).

6. Michael F. Jacobson, *Eater's Digest* (Garden City: Doubleday, 1972).

7. General Accounting Office, 1987.

8. *Consumer Life* Winter 1982.

9. Martha Wagner, "Supermarkets Get Health Smart," *Good Food* September 1987.

10. Wagner.

11. Sources: U.S. Department of Agriculture; and manufacturers (1987).

19. *How to Cure a Sweet Tooth*

1. Holly Hall, "Tired? Take a Walk," *Psychology Today* May 1987.

2. "Eating Fresh Fruit Can Reduce Risk of Stroke," Associated Press, January 29, 1987.

3. "Grapefruit Pectin Reduces Cholesterol," *Science News* 25 July 1987.

4. Jane E. Brody, *Jane Brody's Nutrition Book* (New York: Bantam, 1982).

5. "Apples, A Special Report," *University of California, Berkeley Wellness Letter* May 1989.

6. USDA Human Nutrition Information Service, *Report of the Dietary Guidelines Advisory Committee on the Dietary Guidelines for Americans* 10 Apr. 1985.

7. USDA, *Report.*

Bibliography

Bennett, William, M.D., and Joel Gurin. *The Dieter's Dilemma*. New York: Basic Books, 1982.

Brody, Jane. *Jane Brody's Nutrition Book*. New York: Bantam, 1982.

Center for Science in the Public Interest. *Creative Food Experiences for Children*. Washington, D.C., 1986.

Cheraskin, E. and W. M. Ringsdorf, Jr. *Psychodietetics*. New York: Bantam, 1976.

Cleave, T. L. *The Saccharine Disease: The Master Disease of Our Time*. New Canaan: Keats, 1974.

Crook, William G., M.D. *The Yeast Connection*. New York: Vintage, 1986.

Dufty, William. *Sugar Blues*. New York: Warner, 1976.

Ewald, Ellen Buchman. *Recipes for a Small Planet*. New York: Ballantine, 1973.

Fredericks, Carlton. *Nutrition Guide for the Prevention and Cure of Common Ailments and Diseases*. New York: Simon, 1981.

Hall, Ross Hume. *Food for Nought: The Decline in Nutrition*. New York: Harper, 1974.

Hess, John L., and Karen Hess. *The Taste of America*. New York: Penguin, 1977.

Hunter, B. T. *The Sugar Trap and How to Avoid It*. Boston: Houghton, 1982.

Jacobson, Michael F. *Eater's Digest*. Garden City: Doubleday, 1972.

Lansky, Vicki. *The Taming of the C.A.N.D.Y. Monster*. Wayzata, MN: Meadowbrook, 1978.

Logue, Alexandra. *The Psychology of Eating and Drinking*. New York: Freeman, 1986.

Mariani, John F. *The Dictionary of American Food and Drink*. New York: Ticknor, 1983.

Mayer, Jean. *A Diet for Living*. New York: Pocket Books, 1977.

The New Medicine Show. Mount Vernon, NY: Consumer Reports, 1989.

The Physicians' Manual for Patients. New York: Times Books, 1984.

Stevens, L. J. *The New Way to Sugar Free Cooking*. Garden City: Doubleday, 1984.

Tarr, Yvonne Young. *The New York Times Natural Foods Dieting Book*. New York: Ballantine, 1974.

Trattler, Ross. *Better Health Through Natural Healing*. New York: McGraw, 1985.

Truss, C. O. *The Missing Diagnosis*. Birmingham, AL 35226: (P.O. Box 26508) 1983.

Weiner, Michael A. *Earth Medicine-Earth Food*. London: Collier-Macmillan, 1974.

Yudkin, John, M.D. *Sweet and Dangerous*. New York; Bantam, 1972.

Index